THE FOURTH TRIMESTER COMPANION

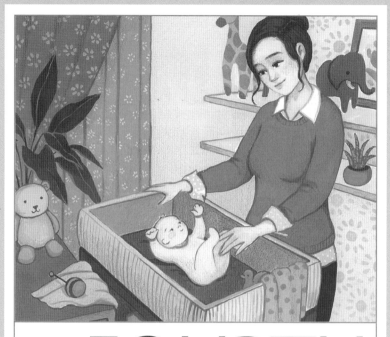

THE FOURTH TRIMESTER COMPANION

HOW TO TAKE CARE OF YOUR BODY, MIND, AND FAMILY AS YOU WELCOME YOUR NEW BABY

CYNTHIA GABRIEL, Ph.D.

HARVARD
COMMON
PRESS

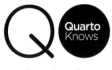

Inspiring | Educating | Creating | Entertaining

Brimming with creative inspiration, how-to projects, and useful information to enrich your everyday life, Quarto Knows is a favorite destination for those pursuing their interests and passions. Visit our site and dig deeper with our books into your area of interest: Quarto Creates, Quarto Cooks, Quarto Homes, Quarto Lives, Quarto Drives, Quarto Explores, Quarto Gifts, or Quarto Kids.

First Published in 2018 by The Harvard Common Press, an imprint of The Quarto Group, 100 Cummings Center, Suite 265-D, Beverly, MA 01915, USA.
T (978) 282-9590 F (978) 283-2742 QuartoKnows.com

The Harvard Common Press titles are also available at discount for retail, wholesale, promotional, and bulk purchase. For details, contact the Special Sales Manager by email at specialsales@quarto.com or by mail at The Quarto Group, Attn: Special Sales Manager, 401 Second Avenue North, Suite 310, Minneapolis, MN 55401, USA.

21 20 19 18   2 3 4 5

ISBN: 978-1-55832-887-7

Digital edition published in 2018

Library of Congress Cataloging-in-Publication Data available.

Design and page layout: Laura H. Couallier, Laura Herrmann Design
Cover Image: Lola and Bek
Photography: Shutterstock.
Illustration: Gayle Isabelle Ford

Printed in China

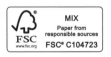

MIX
Paper from
responsible sources
FSC® C104723

The information in this book is for educational purposes only. It is not intended to replace the advice of a physician or medical practitioner. Please see your health-care provider before beginning any new health program.

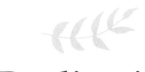

Dedication

This book is dedicated to Diane Scherzer Black and Celeste Craig. Your support, love, patience, and guidance had a profound impact on me, as a mother to Sylvia, Calvin, and Anju. Thank you.

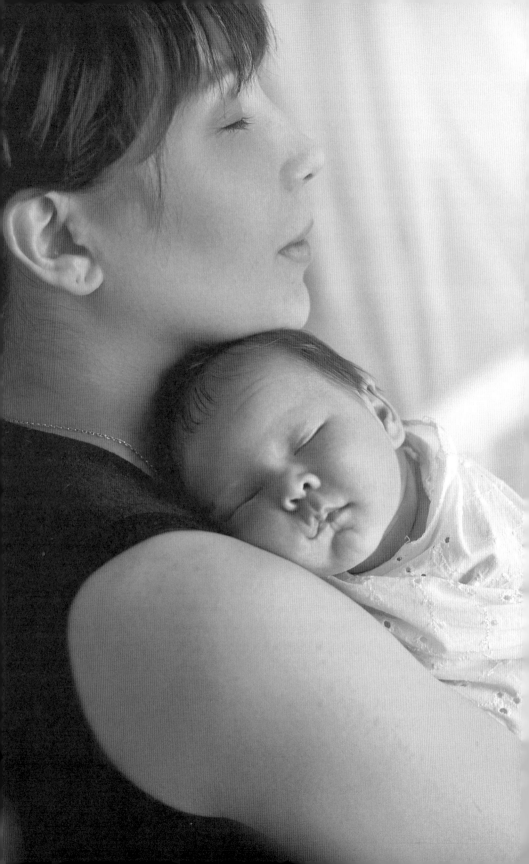

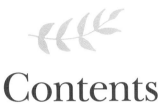

Contents

Introduction

THE FOURTH TRIMESTER IS ONLY THREE MONTHS LONG. In many cultures, intuitive recognition of this special time is built into rituals. New mothers and babies in so many societies are sequestered and cared for in special ways for about forty days. When you are immersed in this time, every day can feel like a year. Simultaneously, when you look back on your first week or your first month with a newborn, you might feel like it happened in a blink. Because it can feel so fast, I think this period is often glossed over in Western culture. A time that deserves much thought and care is, too often, rushed and undervalued.

The "fourth trimester" term came about as a way to recognize that human babies are born extremely needy. Other mammals are born more fully developed than human babies. Think of how baby horses or elephants are able to walk so soon after birth, for example. Researchers who compared the neurological development of newborn chimpanzees and newborn humans found that human babies would have to remain fetuses for up to eighteen months, or *twice as long*, to be born with the same relative brain maturity of chimpanzees at birth. Though anthropologists argue over *why* human babies are born earlier in their development than any other mammal, the fact that human babies are born more helpless is not debated. One theory worth considering during *your* baby's fourth trimester is that human babies need to learn through social interaction more than any other species. That means their need for interaction with *you* is possibly the reason they are born so early.

I invite you to see the fourth trimester as a special time for you and your family. Think of your little one as needing constant care and human touch for the first three months, as if she were still gestating. It doesn't mean every moment will be blissful, but my experience with hundreds of new mothers indicates that the more mindfully and slowly you return to "regular life" after having a baby, the more bliss you are able to feel.

The work of mothering, and fathering, is slow-paced and repetitive. As I explain in chapter 1 (see page 13), parenting challenges can be measured in hours, while joy is usually measured in moments. To be a parent we have to develop the ability to listen carefully, even to small humans who cannot yet speak words. We live with a dichotomous understanding of time as something both infinite and limited. On one hand, we sit with two-year-olds crying about losing their blanket as if this is truly the most momentous calamity; on the other, we are well aware of work deadlines blinking on our computer calendars.

This book is designed to help you stop and pay attention—in the moment. I wanted to write a book that focused on the experience of the birthing mother as she recovers and changes in the immediate postpartum period and learns how to be a parent. Many books focus exclusively on baby care and development, when, in reality, parents also experience a life transition. You are becoming a new person when you add or expand the role of "mother."

Most of this book appears as a rational guide to self-care and baby care in the fourth trimester. However, I hope that underneath the advice and tips sprinkled throughout these pages, you also glimpse the veneration and appreciation I hold for the work you are doing. I have spent a great deal of my professional life in the presence of babies being born. By nature, I am a rational thinker; by professional experience, I have become a mystic. I find the experience of witnessing childbirth to be transcendental and numinous.

As a new mother, when I encountered someone who really understood what I was going through, I felt *seen*. Until those moments, I did not even know I had felt invisible. But, for much of my parenting life, I, like so many others, have indeed felt invisible. I am grateful for all those who held me up as a mother, helped me develop skills, and gave me permission to enjoy this time in the cycle of life.

By consciously gathering the wisdom of those who have gone before me or who have walked next to me into this book, I hope to contribute to your sense of self-respect and confidence in parenting. What you are doing in this sphere is equally worthy of discussion, study, and being shared as any other part of your life. I want to live in a society in which the reproductive and productive work we do are equally valued. When both sides of this equation are balanced, I think we all feel better and treat each other with more kindness and respect than we do when one side is more esteemed than another.

I also wish to impart the immense value of *being supported* in your parenting efforts. Unfortunately, it is possible to parent in a virtual vacuum, just taking care of your children the best you can without much input from anyone else. I fear that this is the default mode of Western parenting.

I accidentally discovered how wonderful it is to feel supported in parenting when one of my children was diagnosed with autism. When my neurotypical children were between two and five years old, my husband and I were, basically, on our own to muddle through parenting dilemmas. Our own parents lived far away. We frequently moved to new cities for our work. I survived by communing with other mothers of young children. (Here's looking at you Tracey Reid, Lavetta Griffin, Alex Vamos, and Jennifer Woodill!)

By contrast, when my child on the autism spectrum was between two and five years old, I had an army of experts whom I could consult for advice and support. I benefitted from professionals who came into my house, observed how I parented, and offered advice. Not everyone welcomes this particular form of support, but, for me, it was positive and life changing. My parenting was *visible* in a novel way, and I learned to accept support in new ways.

That experience has taught me I can reach out much, much more than I previously believed I could. While some of those professionals are paid, many volunteered their time and expertise. Now, for virtually any parenting challenge I face, I feel empowered to reach out for advice and support. Some stalwart friends are there most of the time; others offer support during a short phase of my life. In turn, I give to new parents where I can. In business, this is called "networking." In parenting, it is "community." The difference networking can make to your career is huge; the difference community can make to your family life is incalculable.

I wish you a joyous fourth trimester as you care for yourselves and your newborns. Smell their beautiful newborn scent and bask in the way they trust the Universe to care for them. *You* are their universe for now. You have never been more important.

....

Writing Notes:

A few notes are warranted to help you understand some of what is written here. I have changed the names of all the mothers and fathers who shared their stories with me, although I maintained the names of their real hometowns. However, with permission, I retained the real names of all the birth professionals who contributed to this book, even if they shared a personal story.

I have alternated the pronouns "she" and "he" throughout the book, unless specifically retelling a story of a particular baby girl or boy.

Another language issue arises in that some people who have given birth are male, transgender, or nongendered. Without a more inclusive solution at the time of writing this book, I chose feminine words (she, her, woman, mother) to refer to "mothers." Because I care about the content of this book reaching as many people who need it as possible, I err on what I believe is the wrong side of history. I hope what is useful can reach those people who need it despite the inadequacy of language to address the real diversity of experience. I am looking forward to a changed society in the near future.

Overall, my intention is to cultivate a supportive attitude toward all parents, including parents who have beliefs different from my own. As a doula, I have supported birthing families who espoused many beliefs I do not share, and I am glad for those experiences. Whether you are Christian, Hindu, Jewish, Muslim, atheist, or profess some other faith, the experience of parenting is humbling and exhausting. Parents everywhere can benefit from support and encouragement. Support can come from unlikely sources. As an anthropologist, I have witnessed many diverse cultures. I have learned that being open and curious creates connections. I wish we could all offer that curiosity and openness to each other, so all parents feel valued in the work they do.

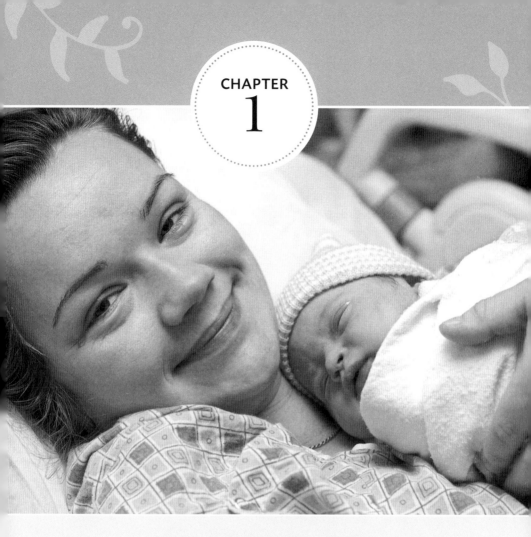

WELCOME TO
THE FOURTH TRIMESTER:
BLISSFUL MOMENTS,
CHALLENGING HOURS

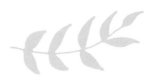

YOU ARE SNUGGLED IN BED (OR ON THE COUCH) with a beautiful, incredibly soft bundle that fits just so in your arms. When your baby is asleep, you rub your cheeks across her wispy hair and it feels like those clouds in paintings of angels. You're eager for everyone you know to meet this little human. You've never felt closer to your partner than you have since this baby was born. Although other people's babies are often wrinkly and ugly, surprisingly, yours is cute and adorable from the get-go. This is what you were waiting for all those months of pregnancy! It feels like a dream come true.

On the other hand, your breasts are as hard as rocks and three times bigger than any bra you own. When your baby is awake, she cries constantly and wants to be bounced. You are afraid to stand up because there could be a red stain on the sheets and you don't want to do another load of laundry. You haven't slept a full night since before you went into labor and that was six days ago. Your partner's mother wants to meet the baby, but you wish she would come back next year. To make matters worse, your partner just made a suggestion about the baby that feels insensitive and unsupportive. It is a nightmare.

Both paragraphs describe the first week with a newborn, probably for the same woman on the same day.

Note: This chapter is about being *home* postpartum with a newborn. If your baby is in the NICU (neonatal intensive care unit), this chapter will probably be more useful to you *after* you get home, or after a few weeks have passed and you are able to focus more on issues besides your baby's health. Feel free to skip directly to "NICU Families" (see page 41). Come back to these earlier chapters as they feel relevant to you.

All of this is normal. It is absolutely okay that not every minute of the first weeks of your baby's life is about transcendent love and ecstasy. If you can believe the difficult moments are just as normal and necessary as the delightful moments, you will come out of this fourth trimester with more stamina and reserves for the months ahead. Fighting the reality or beating yourself up just leads to exhaustion.

My experience as a doula means I have visited many women in the first weeks after giving birth. I have also interacted with hundreds of new mothers in postpartum support groups. The most common theme I hear is a mother's guilt about not enjoying the first weeks "enough." New parents often cry as they describe the reality of their experience. But the guilt they feel is built on an expectation that the first weeks with a new baby are supposed to be easy, fun, and blissful. I am here to tell you they rarely are and, what's more, they are not supposed to be. They are fun and blissful—in moments—but those moments are parts of a larger picture in which the hours may not be enjoyable at all. You are in the fourth trimester and it is a lot of work.

If this is your first baby, you are on an enormously steep learning curve. The curve does not plateau for about three or four months. That is why cultures all over the world give new mothers approximately forty days to recover from birth. It is not so they can stare into their babies' eyes with love and devotion. It is so they can ride the roller coaster of hormones and emotions that occur in those weeks, recuperate from the physical exertion of labor, recover from pregnancy, learn how to breastfeed, and sync their sleeping schedules to their babies' instead of the clock. This work is so demanding that new mothers across the globe are usually protected from the vagaries of everyday life. They are not expected to cook, clean, wash clothes, or stay up-to-date on the news.

The Emotions, Joys, and Worries of the First Week

The hurricane of emotions does have a few predictable ups and downs. In Western culture, we often talk about the baby's "growth spurts" as the reason for new behaviors that require shifts in the new parents. We rarely discuss our own growth spurts, which occur on the physical, mental, emotional, and spiritual levels. But there are a few times when we can say with some certainty that the mother's hormones are shifting and her body is changing in ways we can predict. These shifts are usually accompanied by heightened emotional sensitivity. The chart here describes a few times you might expect some highs and lows. In this chapter, I focus on the emotions and experiences of the first week.

MAMA MILESTONES	WHAT YOU MIGHT FEEL
The first two hours after your baby is born vaginally or the first hours after you recover from cesarean anesthesia	Emotional high
Three to five days after giving birth	Intense highs and lows, often the lowest you have felt since giving birth
About six weeks	Emotional leveling out, a growing confidence that starts to build
About twelve weeks	Often a sense that a "baby fog" is lifting; you feel more interest and engagement in the larger world; usually coincides with a baby's growing interest in toys/objects and learning to control his own hands and feet. This allows parents some breathing room they did not have before, when the baby was not interested in anything but being held, bounced, or fed.

First Two Hours After a Baby Is Born: Emotional High Point

Your Physical and Emotional State

Your body is naturally wired to be awake and aware for about two hours after your baby is born. You are primed to bond strongly with your baby and, often, with your partner immediately after giving birth. Strong, positive emotions usually flood through you as you experience the triumph of birthing your baby (and it is a triumph no matter how it happens—your baby has transitioned from your womb to the world) and the joy of beholding your new child. You are likely to make meaningful and lasting memories in these two hours. Then you and your baby will usually fall into a deep sleep of recovery.

An important caveat: Bonding is not a one-time event!

Our understanding of this sensitive bonding time has increased considerably over the past few years. More and more studies confirm that mammals, including humans, are primed for these moments in a special way. Care providers are increasingly aware and respectful of these sacred family moments. Many hospitals routinely keep mothers and babies together and perform exams and procedures while the baby is with the mother. That does not mean that it's always possible to have your baby with you for these first two hours. It's important to keep in mind that humans are complex.

If you feel like you missed out on bonding in the immediate postpartum period, don't worry! We continue to have a flood of the bonding hormones for a long time postpartum, and humans are quite able to bond by creating the right conditions for it. In fact, we know that men who experience skin-to-skin contact with newborns and care for infants start to release more oxytocin (the cuddling and "love" hormone) and less testosterone and that this happens continuously over time. Pam Belluck writes in the *New York Times*, "Testosterone, that most male of hormones, takes a dive after a man becomes a parent. And the more he gets involved in caring for his children —changing diapers, jiggling the boy or girl on his knee, reading *Goodnight Moon* for the umpteenth time—the lower his testosterone drops." Bonding is not a one-time deal.

In addition, we are different from other mammals in that we can create hormone releases through thinking about events or people who are not even present. Unlike other mammals, human parents can experience the benefits of increased oxytocin just by thinking about their baby. No matter how difficult the immediate postpartum period may have been, you will be able to love and parent your baby well.

How This Plays Out This is usually a high point full of strong, happy, bonding emotions. Women and their partners, even after long, exhausting labors, get a surge of energy. Babies are usually wide-awake, too, looking directly at the parents' eyes and toward their voices. Babies will lick the mother's nipples and latch on (or make great efforts to do so) in these first two hours before sleepiness sets in. If your baby is able to smell and lick your breasts, even without a successful latch, it is a great beginning! This helps her orient to you and the new world she has entered which will, for several months, revolve around your breasts.

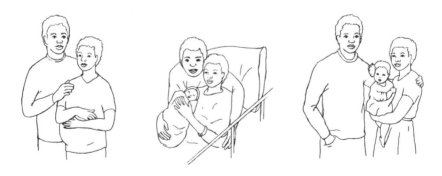

Licking your nipples helps the baby acquire helpful bacteria for her gut and also initiates complex communication between your body and the baby's. We believe our babies are able to make special requests of your mammary glands through saliva, such as, "Please make milk higher in germ-fighting elements because I am exposed to a cold." This communication can begin moments after birth.

Vaginal Birth with Immediate Skin-to-Skin Contact

Mothers can usually remember these moments with clarity—and certainly better than they tend to remember labor. Jessica, a mother of three, relates that, "I feel like there are snapshots from the first hours of my children's lives that are clearer than almost anything else. I did not know I was making such strong memories at the moment, but they are there, indelibly printed on me. If I lose my memory later in life like my grandmother did, I think I'll still always remember my little babies."

Thinking of the high moments as "snapshots" is a helpful tool for this early postpartum period. Recognizing small moments that are tender and dear (and often short in duration) will help you later with the more challenging hours.

Although the placenta is born, perineal tears are evaluated and possibly repaired, and people push on your uterus in ways that feel unexpectedly painful, most women do not remember these physical aspects of the first two hours very vividly. The baby usually takes center stage.

Cesarean Birth

Mothers who give birth by cesarean section are increasingly insisting on skin-to-skin contact and early breastfeeding with their babies as soon as they are born. Still, there is often more separation between mother and baby in this situation than with a vaginal birth. It is helpful to empower the partner to be a vocal go-between, someone who can give running commentary to the mother about what is happening with the baby.

It is absolutely worth it to bring a doula into the operating room, if at all possible, who can play this role for both parents, helping them stay calm, more connected to the baby, and more aware of what is happening. This may require advance negotiation with your medical team so they know your desire in the event of a cesarean, or it can be accomplished by strong insistence from the mother and/or her partner at the time in labor when cesarean birth is being decided.

When I am a doula at a C-section, I focus on communicating the kind of news that helps the new mother feel connected to her baby. Instead of describing what the nurses or doctors are doing or what the medical concerns are, I describe the baby: "Oh, it looks like he has a lot of hair!" or, "His hands are in little fists and they are so cute and tiny!"

Vaginal or Cesarean Birth when Your Baby Is Separated from You

If your baby has trouble breathing at first or has another health concern, your heightened awareness at this time can bring a lot of fear. Especially at a birth, when all the people in the room are focused on the baby and no one is focused on the mother's feelings, this natural "high point" can become a difficult memory. I try to help women for whom the first two hours were not beautiful, "get-to-know-you" moments, see their worry for what it is: bonding. All that fear is really love expressed toward your baby. You will be able to access that same deep love as you move forward.

Advice for the First Two Hours

Because mother and baby tend to fall asleep after about two hours, parents who are prepared may feel like they were better able to focus on their first acquaintance with their baby. Here are some ideas to keep in mind:

- Plan ahead for this time. Whose job will it be to focus on the mother's experience? This is especially important if your baby is whisked away to the warmer across the room or to the NICU.

- Plan to have your baby with you, skin to skin. Your partner might also want to remove clothes for skin-to-skin contact with the baby. Your body temperature will help your baby stay warm.

- The white, lotion-like cream on your baby's skin is called "vernix." Although you will probably wipe away blood and amniotic fluid from your baby with a baby blanket, the vernix is best rubbed into your baby's skin and into yours. It's nature's perfect skin lotion.

- Under normal conditions, all baby tests can be performed while the baby is on you and everything else can be safely delayed.

- Do not set goals about achieving a first latch immediately, although putting your baby to your breast early is a great idea. It's okay if your baby latches and it's okay if your baby sniffs and licks and bobs around. These are important steps toward latching and breastfeeding as well.

First Two Days: Before Your Milk Comes In

If your baby is healthy and with you, more or less, all the time in these first two days, you are likely to be in a relatively steady emotional state as you move between sleep and wakefulness. Breastfeeding may come easily or may come with challenges.

Your Physical and Emotional State

Though you may be working on challenges that develop in the first two days, they rarely rise to the level of "serious concern" so quickly. Catch up on your sleep as much as you can. Offer your baby your breast whenever she fusses.

In the first days, your breasts produce colostrum, which is yellowish and thick. Colostrum is wonderful for your baby's health and immune system. It has more immunity-building properties (such as antibodies and leukocytes) than regular breast milk. As colostrum is, literally, the first food to reach your baby's digestive tract, it has the important job of "sealing" the permeable newborn intestines. There is not nearly as much colostrum as there will be milk (in a few days), so expect your baby to lose some weight at first. The rule of thumb is that babies can lose about 10 percent of their original weight—a little more if you received fluids through an IV during labor—without any worry.

What You Might Notice about Your Baby

Your baby is likely to be very sleepy in the first days. Newborns are used to being held tightly in your womb space. You will notice newborns startle easily, even in their sleep, because there is so much more room in the world than they are used to. In many cultures, babies are swaddled tightly because this helps them stay calm. You can do this even more naturally by holding your baby tightly against your naked body with a blanket on top of you both for warmth. Later, babywearing will also help your baby feel safe.

Baby fingernails are generally quite long at birth and require a trim within the first week. If you are not at home and did not pack baby fingernail scissors (which I always found easier than fingernail clippers), use socks as mittens to protect your baby's face from scratches.

Your baby's head may seem elongated, which is normal after birth (even a cesarean birth, if your baby was low in your pelvis). If it bothers you, put a hat on her head—this is usually camouflage enough. The swelling will go down in just a few days.

You will probably notice your baby's genitalia seem disproportionately large. This swelling is because your hormones have been shared with your baby. In a few weeks or months, the proportions even out. Girl babies can sometimes have vaginal discharge, even blood, which will go away as your hormones leave her body. Some babies, girls and boys, have swelling around their nipples and can even produce a milky liquid. Again, this is normal and ends quickly.

What You Will Notice about Your Body

You will bleed for several weeks after giving birth, whether you gave birth vaginally or by cesarean. As time goes by, the bleeding gradually slows. This gradual slowing—and change from bright red blood to darker red and brown, and even white discharge—is the normal course. Midwives the world over are known for telling mothers that if they suddenly get more bright red blood after the first few days, it is an indication they are doing too much. It is a beautiful, natural way for your body to remind you to slow down. If there is more than just a little bright red blood, though, consult your caregiver. My doula partner, Martha Baum, waxes poetic to all new mothers about the extremely comfortable, but admittedly unfashionable, hospital mesh underwear. If you had a homebirth, according to Martha, order some anyway.

For soreness in the perineal area, try cold packs and witch hazel pads. These help many women feel better. A bag of frozen peas is just the right size and more flexible than ice packs. Of course, don't put anything frozen directly on your skin; use a towel to protect your tender tissue.

Going to the bathroom may feel like a superhuman feat. Functions you have taken for granted suddenly take effort and may be painful. For the most part, this soreness slowly and gradually resolves itself. Your urethra and anus are not accustomed to large, hard objects pushing against them for hours. They are probably bruised and pushed out of shape, and there may be tears or stitches nearby. Women who have tears or skid marks often feel a stinging sensation when they urinate. In this case, use a handheld squeeze bottle to wash your perineal area, which is gentler to these tissues than wiping.

For many mothers, the *thought* of passing a bowel movement after giving birth is worse than the reality. For some women, of course, having a bowel movement is not a big deal. For others, it is. It can be painful, especially if you become constipated. Drink, drink, drink! You will have exerted the muscles of your perineal area during any pushing you did, so it makes sense that these muscles are sore. A few days makes a world of difference in this area.

Your care providers will push on your abdomen in a deep and, often, painful manner for the first days after you give birth. They are checking to see how small your uterus is and giving it a little massage to help it contract. If you don't know about this ahead of time, it can be disconcerting. You might have thought the painful parts were behind you. Mothers who have given birth more than once can also experience painful contractions for a few days postpartum as the uterus devolves.

If pain accompanies your bathroom trips for more than a week or two, or if it is more intense than feels manageable, talk to your care provider. Occasionally, women need more than just time to heal their perineum. In France, the state medical system pays for all women to undergo what they call "perineal re-education" to firm up musculature and prevent incontinence. Although the first week is a time to rest and recover, not actively work out, most women *can* benefit from perineal exercise at around six weeks postpartum.

Advice for the First Two Days

I urge you to cultivate calm and let others worry about routine baby health issues. In the first twenty-four to forty-eight hours, medical personnel are looking for jaundice (relatively common) and for many other rare, but important, issues. They check to make sure, for example, your baby can metabolize the amino acid phenylalanine and does not have cystic fibrosis. It is easy to get swept up into a feeling of anxiety, especially if labor was long or involved scary elements. Just because the medical personnel have to be worried about everything going wrong with you and your baby, does not mean you have to be!

Many new mothers arrive home a day or two after giving birth particularly panicked about two issues in particular:

- The baby is not eating enough.
- The baby has jaundice.

I wish there were a way to help more mothers feel calm about these two matters. It's important to be alert to potential problems, but, because these usually resolve by themselves within a few days, it is not worth the fear so many mothers experience. Cultivate your own feeling of calm however you can. Surround yourself with calm people, such as a doula or experienced mother. If there really is a health issue, be confident you will find it and handle it appropriately. There is no need to worry in advance. Let the midwives, nurses, and doctors do that for you.

Day Three (Four, or Five): Intense Ups and Downs

Between Day Three and Day Five, usually culminating in one terrible day, most new mothers experience a dip in their emotional state. Be forewarned: This dip is often dramatic.

Your Physical and Emotional State

Whereas a woman might have been enjoying the bond with her new baby in the first two to three days, she may experience strong feelings of despair and regret around the third or fourth day. For others, it is less dramatic, but still noticeable.

The cause of this emotional dip is a perfect storm of ingredients. You have the potent combination of changing hormone levels interacting with lack of sleep on the physical side of the equation. On the mental side, you are starting to see the reality of what it means to be responsible for another human being's welfare twenty-four hours a day, every day, without a break. And you also have a pediatrician telling you, "It's probably nothing, but you should keep your eye on X and Y."

If you've ever stayed awake all night, you know there can be a high the next day that allows you to push through another sleepless period. But it can't last. Eventually, you crash. If your labor was long and caused you to miss sleep, or your baby and nurses kept waking you up the first two nights after you gave birth (or both!), you will have exhausted your sleep reserves by the third day after delivery. That's enough to make anyone grouchy and upset!

But that sleep deprivation is also combined with massive shifts in hormone levels. After the incredible high of giving birth and meeting your new baby, which is associated with elevated levels of oxytocin (the "love" hormone) and endorphins (the "runner's high" hormone), it makes sense there will be a crash. Even if your body just produces a little bit less oxytocin or endorphins, it will feel like a descent. Other hormones (progesterone, prolactin, relaxin, etc.), also shift rapidly in this immediate postpartum period to change your body from a pregnant body to a lactating body.

Combine all these physical challenges with the experience of the first two or three days of your baby's life. It was fun, at first, to try to figure out how to soothe your crying baby. It was amazing, at first, to see your newborn latch on to your breast and suck as if she always knew how. It was a happy moment when you woke in the middle of the first night to snuggle your infant who was making loud snorting sounds in her sleep. But around Day Three or Day Four, many women (especially of first babies) start to project this reality forward. *Having a baby who cries whenever I am not holding him means I will never have two empty arms again!*

In addition to all this, these first days present many parenting roadblocks. You might be experiencing breastfeeding challenges, and getting conflicting advice about how to handle them. Your pediatrician

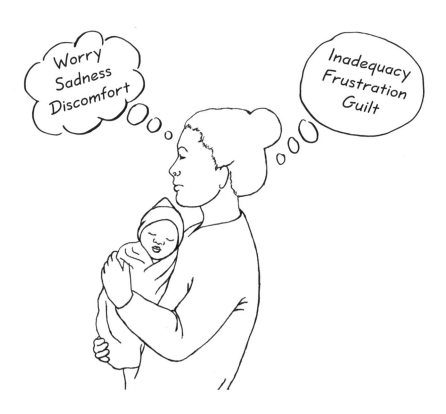

has probably scheduled a baby checkup for one of these days. You will have to get yourself and your baby dressed, pack a diaper bag, and brave your car or public transit to get to your doctor's office.

Then, if you are like most families, you will be told to be vigilant about your baby's weight loss/gain and your baby's color. As I've already noted, most babies lose weight in the first few days postpartum and it takes a while for babies to start to regain their birth weight and then surpass it. In the meantime, the pediatrician and you hold your breath with some anxiety as you wait to see if your baby is following this pre-dictable pattern or if something else is going on.

Many, many babies are considered a little jaundiced. Admittedly, jaundice is important to treat if it becomes a real issue, but usually it does not. Normally, jaundice resolves on its own through breastfeeding, your baby's bowel movements, and sunlight exposure. It can easily become just another pointless worry to add to the overwhelming list of new worries for average parents. What you can do is spend time out-doors during sunlight hours (bundled up, if necessary, with face and hands exposed) and breastfeed as much as you can.

In sum, you might experience all or some of these things on this "Flood Day:"

- Continued pain from episiotomy repairs or tears
- Painfully engorged breasts
- Annoyance at laundry needs from bleeding and leaking milk
- Crying (both you and baby)
- Backward progress on baby's latch because your breasts are so engorged
- Sadness (even despair)
- Feelings of inadequacy
- Feelings of powerlessness
- Worry about your baby's health
- Worry that your baby is not getting enough milk or nutrients
- Worry that your baby is jaundiced
- Desire for a break, or to run away

- Anger, annoyance, or guilt toward loved ones such as parents or in-laws
- Guilt
- Despair about ever being yourself again
- Possible sadness about how your postpartum body looks or feels
- Stress about life's logistics (i.e., making dinner or a trip to the pediatrician)
- Worry about an older child's adjustment to a sibling

When you add all this up, it is amazing that we ask a cute baby to balance this scale. Of course, when our hormones recalibrate, cute babies generally do balance it, which just shows you how powerful babies are.

I am here to tell you: This is all normal. And it will pass. In fact, it rarely lasts more than a day or two. Somehow, we regroup and adjust to the new hormones and new experiences. I asked my doula friends to name this day and these were the suggestions I received:

- Stuff-Gets-Real Day
- Leaking-Out-of-Every-Hole-in-My-Body Day
- The-Milk-Hits-the-Fan Day
- Lactifuddlement
- Bring It On!!! Day
- Milk Overwhelm/Milk Adjustment/Milk Transition
- Mother Hazing
- The Humbling and Let It Go
- The Universal Shift
- The Blow Out
- The Big Bust
- The Flood
- Hormone Leap Day
- Milk Tears

Give this day your own name and share it with me. I'd like to bring more awareness to this experience among pregnant mothers and a good name would be helpful. Whatever you call it, it's a transition that involves *all* your feelings.

Advice for This Messy Day

Knowing this may occur may make it feel less intense. Forewarned is forearmed. Mothers, you need your very best, most supportive friend to visit you on this day. Send your other friends out to buy you comfort food and maybe a soft robe that zips up the front (very useful for breastfeeding), but do not let anyone into the house who cannot handle your full emotional range. If you had a birth doula, it's a great idea to schedule a postpartum visit for around Day Four or Five.

Do not invite your mother or mother-in-law over unless you have a strong relationship built on support and trust. Anyone likely to feel a need to rescue you or your baby should not be invited over, because what you really need on this "Messy Day" is someone to listen and love you. There isn't too much more to be done.

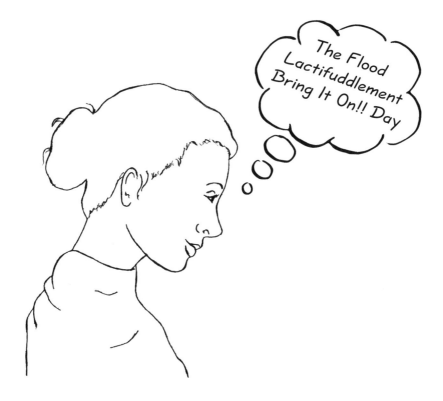

The First Week for Partners

Mom and baby are the "main show"—as they should be. But you, the mother's chosen partner, are still a vital part of a successful first week. You may have been at your partner's side through labor and delivery and, like many partners, you may have felt helpless to do anything. If you ask, however, you are likely to hear, "She couldn't have done it without you." Your presence is more valuable than you know.

There is a lot you can do to support your partner in these first weeks. If she is breastfeeding, arrange her pillow supports and get her a drink of water (with a straw is helpful) when she's ready to nurse. Take over specific chores, such as diaper changes or baby baths. If you do this, you are assured of special bonding time with your baby and your partner is assured of mini time-outs from baby care. Make a point of giving your partner time to herself. A shower and a half-hour to relax can do wonders for her mood.

If there is any way you can afford to stay home and be part of the two-week cocoon, I urge you to do so. The first two weeks present a steep learning curve for new parents. It's best to go through that together, if possible. If you have older children, even more reason to stay home. They will benefit from more attention at this time, too.

Just as new birth mothers have to take care of themselves while they take care of a baby, so do you! If you are able to engage in activities that your partner cannot, such as going out with friends in the evening or going for a run, I urge you to do so after the first few weeks at home. It's helpful, however, to acknowledge—aloud—that you understand your partner might also wish to do those things. That acknowledgment can go a long way toward heading off resentment.

Lesbian partners and fathers also experience hormonal shifts through the act of caring for a newborn. Skin-to-skin contact with infants makes us all release more oxytocin, the cuddling and love hormone.

Here are the voices from some partners about their experiences in the first weeks of living with a baby.

Jerome: *I knew it was going to be the "Alice-and-Jackson" show as soon as we got home from the hospital, but I had no idea how bad I would feel about it. It felt like a bad dream, where you are standing outside the dance club in line and they can't find your name on the invite list, but you know all your friends are inside. I felt totally outside. Just not part of what was happening. I served food and answered emails. Alice's friends came over to see the baby, and it was like I didn't even exist. I don't think Alice had any idea how excluded I felt. It took a long time before it felt like we were a family and I was part of it.*

Larissa: *My wife already had one child from a previous relationship, so I had a ready-made family when we got married. But this was my first baby. Theresa (my wife) knew how to do everything, of course, so I felt a bit like a third wheel. Fourth wheel, really. I'm not proud of this, but I ended up working even more than I usually do. It made Theresa really mad, but I am paid for every client I see, and making money was the only thing I felt capable of doing right then. Things didn't turn around until Theresa got a really bad flu. That was about five weeks after she came home from the hospital. That was when I first felt like I stepped up and figured out how to be a parent. Theresa slept and, even though she was still nursing, I was doing everything else. After that, I felt more confident, like I had something to offer besides money.*

Marco: *So, I was really focused on the car seat. I look back now—it was a little obsessive. I wanted to do something to take care of our baby. So I obsessed about the car seat. But now that Lika is three, I look back at how scared I was to actually hold her. If she cried, I pretty much gave her back to my wife. Those first few weeks were just scary. Lika cried, my wife cried, and I had no idea what to do. My wife is pregnant and I'm glad I get a chance to re-do it. Now I love hanging out with my daughter, but I just didn't know how to do that at first.*

Andrew: *After our baby was born, my wife was in the hospital for three months because of a bad reaction to her epidural. She was temporarily paralyzed and couldn't walk. So, I was the main parent. I took care of Neveah by myself for almost three months. My parents came to help, but they are a lot older and couldn't really help at night. I was surprised at how natural it all felt. If Neveah cried, I just figured out what she wanted. Her needs were so basic: eat, change her diaper, hold her. She loved to be held! At first, I just stared at her, but after a few weeks, I was able to hold Neveah and read the paper. I've never been so caught up on the news.*

As a visual person, I sometimes find pictures communicate more than words. It's worth taking the time to explore positive representations of parents beyond just images of birth mothers. Here are two of my favorite sites. For beautiful photos of self-identified "butch" women with babies, visit Butchesandbabies.com. For a powerful visual homage to the role of "father," visit Johan Bävman's website, www.johanbavman.se/swedish-dads. He photographed Swedish fathers with their children in everyday situations.

Your partner may have been an excellent support before, during, and after the birth of your baby. On this day, though, your partner is probably in a similar boat as you: exhausted and overwhelmed. That best girlfriend who is coming over to help you out? Make sure she finds something rejuvenating for your partner to do. Sleep would be the best option, if needed. Also good is a walk around the neighborhood, a massage, or a dip in a hot tub. This may send the mother into spasms of crying because she cannot easily do any of those things, but it is essential that the partner replenish reserves, too.

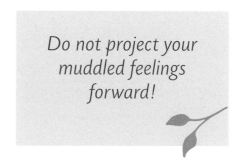

Do not project your muddled feelings forward!

If you are a hot mess in the early days postpartum, do not jump to the conclusion you are experiencing postpartum depression. Culturally, we are quick to interpret this very normal descent as something negative. Women who have had depression in the past may worry it is returning. We are all very sensitive to signs of postpartum depression in new mothers (and in the weeks ahead, do pay attention to signs!). However, in my experience, this normal let down around Day Three is a fluctuation women should interpret as a sign their body is working well.

We are a culture that is especially prone to suppressing emotions and finding it difficult to interpret or even acknowledge complicated emotions. Our extroverted culture leaves little room for introspective feelings such as sadness, disappointment, fatigue, or confusion. Yet these feelings are as real in the postpartum period as joy and wonder. Other cultures support more nuanced understandings of peoples' inner worlds. In Russia, I found that friends, male and female alike, discussed everyday emotions with finely-parsed distinctions. I found Brazilians also prone to talk about deeply-felt experiences such as birth using a wide palette of emotional vocabulary. There was little trouble expressing the "both-and" experience of sadness and happiness.

I have a theory that is impossible to test, but that I share with new mothers. I believe these strong but difficult feelings need to be expressed in some way, if they are there, and suppressing them actually contributes to the development of postpartum depression. Postpartum depression is a complex beast with many contributing factors, including genetics; however, we know social support decreases the incidence and severity of postpartum depression. We also know journal writing and sharing one's feelings with a trusted listener help people who have clinical depression. Based on these studies and my experience with many new mothers, I suspect that accepting our feelings and not fighting them (denying them, telling ourselves we "shouldn't" feel them, etc.), is also important protection. Feel the full range of your feelings on this Flood Day. Then they are able to flow on and away.

Two Weeks a Cocoon, Six Weeks a Nest

The roller coaster of the first five days passes and you enter the "cocoon" phase. My midwife gave me three rules, the top three on this list, which I

Five Rules for New Mothers

1. Wear your pajamas for two weeks (unless it is to go around the block for a short walk).

2. Don't touch money or a credit card for six weeks.

3. Once you are sure your baby is gaining weight, never wake a sleeping baby.

4. Accept all offers of food delivery from people able and willing to leave food at your door without a real visit.

5. Don't worry about creating habits in your baby for the long run.

share with you. I have added two rules out of my experience as a mother and a doula.

You can *change* your pajamas as often as you like, however, said my midwife. And mothers are certainly encouraged to shower or take baths whenever they can. Don't try to wear regular street clothes. Although you may spend a lot of time on your couch or pacing your living room jostling a baby on your shoulder, staying in your pajamas reminds you —and sometimes, more importantly, the people around you—that you are not available for anything beyond taking care of a baby. It's a subtle way to support the creation of a "cocoon" in your home. For two weeks, it does not matter what is happening in the outside world. The stress of bundling your baby into a car seat, packing up all the things your baby might need, and making yourself "presentable" to the world will be manageable soon enough. But for two weeks, you should not worry about the surprisingly difficult getting-out-of-the-house struggle.

In many countries, pediatricians, nurses, or midwives make home visits during these first two weeks to check on mothers and babies.

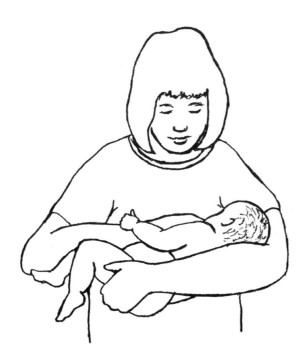

I have a list of issues I would like to see addressed in Canada and the United States, and this is one of the highest on my list! If we are making mothers take babies to pediatrician visits because we care about their health, we should check on the babies at home because that is *better for their health*!

Cooking and cleaning, if possible, should be off the new parents' plates for two weeks (completely) and for six weeks (mostly). This is especially true if you have older children in your home.

Meal Trains

If you have friends or family willing to make meals for you, go out of your way to accept their hospitality. In fact, if no one offers to do this for you, it is an excellent idea to ask a friend to set up a meal train. A meal train is a schedule of meals that friends and family deliver to you. You can decide how often a meal delivery would be useful: every day, every other day, once a week, or some other schedule. New parents can be shy about this, but if you think about how you would feel if a friend or colleague asked you to do this, you will probably see it is an honor and not an imposition. If you have older children, the parents in your older child's class or preschool are often a great resource for meals. If none have offered, it is absolutely fine manners to reach out to one and make a request. Sometimes, a golden parent will also be able to make snacks or lunches for your older children to bring to daycare or school.

There are several wonderful websites that can be used to organize meal trains, including:

- Carecalendar.org
- Mealtrain.com
- Lotsahelpinghands.com
- Takethemameal.com
- Mealbaby.com

If you schedule meals for every other day, you will probably find most people bring large quantities of food that make leftovers. Psychologically, it can also be easier to handle doorstep visitors every other day.

Planning a Meal Train

- Set up your own meal train or ask a friend or relative to set it up for you. Just give the organizer a list of email addresses for inviting.
- State your food preferences up front—or everyone will call to ask! If you give four or five suggestions about foods you like, you'll likely get something good.
- Your meal train organizer can suggest other lovely additions, such as flowers or dessert.
- Suggest take-out utensils and plates, or a specific plan for your meal-makers to pick up used containers. Lots of Tupperware hanging around is not a relaxing sight for new parents.
- Invite everyone you know to participate! Many people are flattered to be included. I've never met someone who felt upset to be asked.
- At least two websites listed previously (see opposite), Carecalendar.org and Lotsahelpinghands.com, let you schedule other things besides meals, such as helping with laundry or babysitting older children. Mealbaby has a feature that allows out-of-town people to buy gift certificates for local restaurants.

The catch is, only invite people to bring you food if they are able to handle *not* being invited inside for a real visit in the first two weeks. This rule should be pinned to the top of the website you use. People seem to respond well to, "We are cocooning with our new baby for two weeks. After that, we are open to short visits!"

Capturing Memories

If you are like most mothers, you will be taking a lot of photos of your newborn. Once you are feeling up to it, which might be right away or months in the future, consider writing down thoughts and memories about your mothering experience and about your baby's milestones. Baby books are increasingly being replaced by more visual, online options, but tactile books can be lovely mementos. I have enjoyed the *Mom's One-Line a Day* books by FastForward Publishing because no matter how tired I am, I can write one sentence. This becomes a book of memories about day-to-day life rather than just the typical milestones.

Although there is great benefit in the typical way we celebrate a baby growing, with photos of first smiles, first teeth, and first steps, there is also value in writing about your experience as a new mother. Young children will like to see the photos of their own growing-up, but adult children will likely someday appreciate insight into your life as a new mother. You can do something like the "sentence-a-day" book electronically. Apps such as "Day One," "Moment Garden," or the online journal Tinybeans are popular. You can spend hours on these if you want to, but you can also just write a little bit when you have an extra minute.

Your Birth Story

Processing and integrating your birth experience begins virtually the moment the experience is over. Women think about their baby's birth for the rest of their lives. Unlike other memories, the memory of your birth experience is likely to take shape in the first week postpartum and remain with you in form and meaning with little revision through your lifetime. Birth expert Penny Simkin found that women's memories of childbirth are "vivid and deeply felt" and easily and accurately recalled decades later.

An important place to begin, when you process your own birth experience, is the acknowledgement that "a healthy mom and a healthy baby" is NOT the only important outcome. How you *felt* about giving birth is equally as important for your mental health. It is possible to feel grateful for your baby's health and simultaneously upset about what happened during your labor. You deserve to have your own full range of feelings about your baby's birth no matter what the physical outcome was.

Some women feel safe and supported through long, physical ordeals and weeks of NICU. Some women feel traumatized by short, intense labors that lead to a healthy infant. Your story is your story, and it is okay to acknowledge any feelings you have about your birth experience.

In the first week postpartum, you will probably tell your baby's birth story several times to several different audiences. Your best friend and your sister, for example, probably want to hear the in-depth moment-by-moment account. Your boss and co-workers, on the other hand, are probably expecting a breezy, upbeat summary. And your mother-in-law may want to hear some details, but not any that feel too intimate.

But what do *you* need? Most women need to process and think through their birth experience in the first week. You just lived through something that was likely intense, dramatic, and highly meaningful. Like the moment you received a long-awaited piece of mail or email (maybe a college acceptance letter or a job offer), or a heightened experience such as a wedding, giving birth is an event we re-live over and over in our minds.

If you had a doula and feel positively toward her, you may naturally end up talking about how things went at your first postpartum visit. An informal online poll of doulas revealed that most doulas try to visit their clients in the first five days. They say their two main goals are to help new mothers process their birth stories and to check on breastfeeding.

Midwives with whom you have developed a close relationship can also serve this purpose, sometimes in the first week when they are checking you and your baby's health, and sometimes at the six-week checkup. For some women, these routine checkups are all that is needed, and a fifteen-minute conversation is sufficient. But, in my experience, women tend to need more than an hour—really, two or three hours—to talk through their birth experience with a trusted listener.

Positive Birth Stories

If your birth experience was relatively smooth and you generally consider it a positive story, you have the right to process your feelings and tell your story just as much as a woman with a more difficult experience. You may have sad feelings about one aspect of your labor that you can release, even if you found the overall experience empowering. As you know, there are many women who have complicated and difficult stories to tell. When a group of new mothers gets together, sometimes those stories dominate and women with positive stories feel like they should not share. For your own sake, and for the sake of our larger culture, I urge you to share whenever it feels possible to do so. Our culture needs more positive birth stories. And you deserve to be honored as a birthing mother.

Complicated Birth Stories

If your birth experience did not go as you expected and you had to make decisions you wish you did not have to make, making peace with your birth experience is important. Likewise, if you felt shamed, mistreated, or disempowered by caregivers during your labor or delivery, it's important to find some closure and peace.

In your case, you may need to put conscious attention toward this healing. You may need to do research to decide whether you feel like certain interventions were necessary or not. Know there will be time to do this research, even if it is not right now. You may want to write a letter to a care provider (or, in some cases, to a medical or licensure board, or to the hospital administration) to express your thoughts. Probably, this is work for a little bit later than the first week postpartum.

I have known women who wrote such letters years after their baby's birth. What you can do now is invite a dear friend over for an afternoon or evening devoted to talking about what happened. Sometimes, a good talk with a friend is all that is needed. But through this process, or even before, you may realize you want more professional help in the form of a therapist. You do not have to have postpartum depression to visit a therapist. In fact, processing difficult birth experiences is a common use of therapy.

Tell Your Story! For many years, I ran weekly mother–baby groups in my community. Once every eight weeks, our discussion topic would be "birth stories." I loved those days! We lit a candle, which we placed in front of the mother who was speaking, usually as she held or breastfed her infant. Each mother told her story and was witnessed by the rest of the group. Without fail, tears would stream down most of our faces as mother after mother described the way her baby came to Earth. Some stories were uplifting and empowering; others were heartbreaking. But the depth of feeling and a sense that "this mother is so strong!" were always palpable. Your story, whether it is a triumphant VBAC (vaginal birth after cesarean) or a four-day-long induction at thirty-five weeks that led to the NICU, is important to tell. Find a listener worthy of hearing it. Tell your story.

NICU Families

If your baby comes very early, or has a health issue requiring prompt treatment in the NICU, your first weeks or months postpartum have different challenges than those of other parents. All parents need a helping hand here and there to get by; NICU parents can use substantial support at every level, from spiritual to emotional to financial. The experience of taking care of your baby and worrying about your baby's health can be an exhausting and depleting one. Research corroborates this subjective experience; parents of children in the NICU have elevated risk for postpartum depression and PTSD.

Of course, you are worried about your baby's health. But it is important that you take care of yourself, too. Veteran NICU parents shared with me their thoughts and tips for surviving this time optimally.

If You Are Breastfeeding, Get Support Right Away

Gina, from Oakland, California, had a baby who came home from the NICU after 116 days. She found not all staff were supportive of breastfeeding, especially preemies like hers, who could not physically latch on. She got the message that formula was "easier" for the staff. Also, she noticed other families in the NICU were generally "less natural minded" than she was, so she got the impression that breastfeeding was less important to many other NICU families than it was to her.

Her advice: "Find the breastfeeding-friendly staff. Listen to their advice more than the advice of other staff. If you can get them on your side, it will help all around."

She bonded with two nurses she calls "angels" because they went so far out of their way to ensure she was able to maintain a good milk supply in the NICU. Even if you have been discharged, but your baby is in the NICU, you can usually ask for daily consultations with the hospital lactation consultants, sometimes more often, if needed.

You should specifically ask hospital staff to use the breastmilk or colostrum you pump for any feedings when you are not present. The default infant food is often formula. There are refrigerators in the NICU to store breastmilk and a nurse can show you how to label your milk so it can be used even when you are not there.

NICUs vary in the furniture that is available next to your baby's bassinette. To breastfeed comfortably, you may need to ask for a better chair, nursing pillows, blankets, or other supplies. These all exist nearby, so don't hesitate to ask. If you are breastfeeding in the NICU often, these usually end up remaining at "your" place.

If your baby is too young to latch on to your breast or suck properly, you may benefit from assistance in learning how to use a pump and establish your milk supply. If you do not feel confident in how this is going after about three days, call a lactation consultant in your community who works outside the hospital. Although most hospital-based lactation consultants are wonderful, finding an independent international board-certified lactation consultant (IBCLCs) can sometimes offer more, or different, advice that is helpful.

Use Hospital Resources. They Are There to Help You!

Hospitals have a bevy of services that often go unused. You probably have access to most or all the following:

- Hospital chaplains
- Hospital financial advisors
- Hospital lactation consultants
- Hospital mental health professionals
- Hospital patient advocate

- Hospital social workers
- Ronald McDonald House, for overnight accommodations

If you feel overwhelmed, ask friendly NICU staff for advice about how to access services. They should know how to initiate an appointment with a hospital mental health professional, social worker, or chaplain. You will probably have to ask, because NICU staff are so focused on taking care of the babies, they may not think to offer.

Even if you are not religious, consider talking with the hospital chaplain. Generally, chaplains are trained to work with people across a variety of faiths, including the nonreligious. Their approach can be calming and comforting.

Marissa and her wife, Kathleen, in upstate New York, first tried a session with the hospital psychiatrist. They found his approach too clinical. Even though neither is religious, they took the advice of a NICU nurse who recommended talking to the hospital chaplain. Marissa says, "I worried about being judged, because, really, if you asked me, I'd say I'm an atheist. But our meetings with Cassie (the chaplain) were like an oasis of calm at that hospital. She was so empathetic and willing to help us in the real world, outside the walls of the hospital, too. We felt really alone during the whole thing. You know, the NICU is busy all night and all day. It's easy to lose track of time. Cassie helped us get grounded and just feel less scared."

Andy Schreider, a father in Cleveland, was anxious about his son in the NICU and he was also scared of the cost that every day of care was incurring. He was able to negotiate a long-term payment plan and reduced fees by talking directly with a hospital financial advisor. Taking that proactive step helped him feel less overwhelmed during the daunting first weeks of his baby's life.

Find the NICU Rhythm That Feels Right to You

Some parents spend most of their time at the NICU; others visit once a day. Some parents sleep at the hospital; others find they function better if they sleep at home. Almost all wonder if they are making the "right" choice. The right amount of time to spend at the NICU with your baby is as much as you can while taking care of yourself and your primary relationships, such as with a partner or other children. If you are not doing well physically or emotionally, you probably need to step away more often to access additional support and take care of yourself.

Sometimes parents need to go back to work while their baby is in the NICU, and this has an impact on the amount of time they can devote to being with their infant. Working is part of taking care of yourself and your family, including your baby.

The rhythm that works for your heart, body, and other relationships is going to be unique to you. Do not compare yourself to any other NICU family.

Hold and Touch Your Baby as Much as You Can

When my daughter was in the NICU, I remember talking to a nurse across the top of her plastic bassinette and feeling like the space of the bassinette belonged to her, the medical professional. Even with all my training and work with other mothers, it felt transgressive to reach in and touch my own baby's skin.

The NICU is set up as a medical space; however, inside this space it is okay, and even essential, to carve out bonding and caring space. You probably wished this bonding space were your own bed or couch. This matters more to you, though, than it does to your baby. What your baby needs is to feel your body temperature, hear your heartbeat, and smell your skin. Take a deep breath and just touch or hold your baby, even if the medical environment feels uninviting. Providing this skin-to-skin contact is often called "kangaroo care."

Researchers in 2016 looked at data from twenty-one studies (that included more than 3,000 low-birth-weight babies) and found that kangaroo care had many benefits for newborns, including better regulation of body temperature, less risk of hospital-acquired infections, and increased weight and length. Given all these known benefits, it might seem like all hospitals and NICUs would automatically encourage this. The truth is, however, that hospital staff, however well meaning, can be too busy and too concentrated on medical procedures to initiate kangaroo care sessions. Parents often have to ask and insist.

Tammy Twaddle, a nurse in Virginia, reminds parents also provide much of the routine care for their babies in the NICU, such as changing diapers and bathing. She writes, "Doing these things will help with the bonding experience and empower them, knowing they are caring for their little one as much as they can." Even some medical care can be performed by parents. You can ask to be taught various procedures. In some cases, you may have to continue them at home anyway.

Development Questions Will Probably Continue Past NICU

If your child is born significantly before the due date, your questions about development will likely last for a few years. On Facebook and online groups for NICU parents, I notice many posts from parents of two- and three-year-olds. Normal growth and development milestones are different for preemie babies than they are for term babies, and this does not even out for quite a while.

Hopefully, your NICU journey will end with a successful transfer to home and you will easily and comfortably transition into regular life with a newborn. Remember to reach out for help and support even after you are home. The feelings of sadness, anger, and shock that often accompany the NICU journey do not magically dissipate the day you return home. In fact, you may have suppressed them during the emergency and may only feel these emotions when they emerge at home.

Online communities may offer a bridge for you between the intensity of the NICU and the day-to-day concerns of home life. You may need time to integrate these often-intense NICU experiences into your life story. Give yourself permission to return to your normal energy levels and your normal levels of optimism, even if you also have other feelings, too.

Like many parents, I found the NICU experience slightly traumatic. Recovering from that while also being the parent of a newborn was confusing. I often did not know whether what I was thinking or feeling was because I was a new mother or because I was recovering from our NICU experience.

Be gentle with yourself, seek and accept help, and enjoy the moments you can. Hopefully, you will soon be more concerned with what brand of detergent best removes baby poo and how to make time for sex with your partner than with your baby's health.

When you are back on your feet, and it makes sense to do so, consider reaching out to other families in your community who have babies in your local NICU. Many parents find that serving others and being a positive role model helps them feel better about the way their own baby's life began.

Conclusion

Enjoy every moment that is an enjoyable moment! Take photos, if you are a picture person. Write down your thoughts every day—they change so fast and you won't remember what you thought two days ago about being a parent.

But, do not put yourself into a "bliss" guilt vise. It is normal that most of your time taking care of a newborn in the first few weeks feels hard, not wonderful. Be kind to yourself and remember that, in most places in the world, you would be honored and pampered for these first forty days. Say "yes" to any help that brings you relief. Say "no" to any help or visitors that do not. You will survive this time and, someday, you may even reminisce about how precious it was. Hindsight makes this hard job look easier than it actually is.

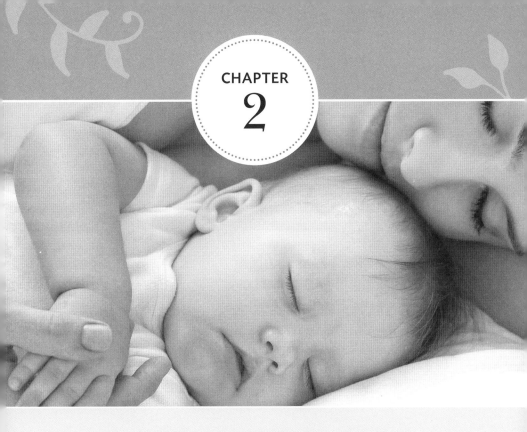

SLEEP: YOUR BABY'S, AND YOURS

Dear New Parent,

Your baby will sleep through the night someday, before he becomes an adult, before he becomes a parent himself and experiences interrupted sleep because of his own baby. Do not worry about how your precious little one is sleeping.

Worry about how you are sleeping! Make sure there is some way for you to get the sleep you need to continue to function and be healthy.

The reason you want your baby to sleep, really, is so you can sleep. Admit this! Accept this! Then move on to find ways to get more sleep for YOU.

Sincerely, An Experienced Mother

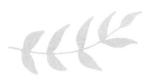

THIS IS THE LETTER I WISH I COULD WRITE to every new parent. I cringe to see all the books (and there are many) that purport to help infants sleep better. Almost all infants have no sleep problems. New parents, on the other hand, often have serious sleep issues.

I do understand the logic at work. The idea is that if you could teach your baby to sleep through the night, then you would be able to sleep through the night. So that does seem like the ideal solution, except that a) it does not work most of the time, and b) it is not the natural way most babies sleep.

> *I am confident your baby will get enough sleep. I am not confident you will.*

There are exceptions. There are a very few babies who naturally sleep for long stretches at night and do so from an early age. I personally know one child, she's much older now, like this. We all marveled at her super-baby skill and felt incredible jealousy toward her mother. As a new parent, I can virtually guarantee you will hear about these exceptions and you will immediately think the exception is the norm and that it is *your* constantly waking baby who is the anomaly.

But, in my experience working with hundreds of new mothers in three countries, I can tell you babies who sleep for many hours at night are definitely in the minority. Most babies wake up a *lot* at night, although they do tend to sleep for longer stretches as they get older. Sleep books that promise to get your baby to sleep either appear to work because, as babies get older, they tend to sleep more (so you'll never know whether it was the advice or your baby just grew out of it), or they won't work at all, in which case parents feel guilty and inadequate. I wade into this subject cautiously, but confident that 99 percent of the time the problem is not with your baby's sleep. It is with *yours*.

Reasons Why Babies Do Not Sleep for Long Stretches

Here are three facts that help explain why babies do not sleep for more than two to four hours at nighttime, normally.

1. A typical newborn's stomach is tiny.

The illustration below shows the size of a newborn's stomach as it grows in the first days and weeks, from approximately the size of a cherry to a large egg. Babies drink a little, digest, and are ready for more soon afterward.

NEWBORN STOMACH SIZE
Why babies need to eat so often.

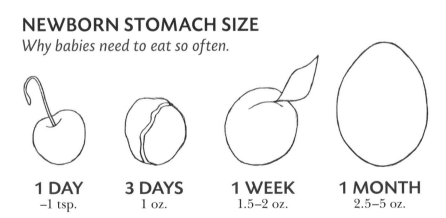

1 DAY	**3 DAYS**	**1 WEEK**	**1 MONTH**
–1 tsp.	1 oz.	1.5–2 oz.	2.5–5 oz.

2. Human breast milk is designed to be drunk often, not just a few times a day.

Some mammals, such as lions or rabbits, nurse their babies and leave them for hours, or even all day, so they can forage for food. These animals produce milk with an extremely high fat content, which takes longer to digest than carbohydrates.

Other mammals, such as chimpanzees and kangaroos, stay with their babies all day and carry them with them everywhere they go. Those babies have constant access to the breast. Animal mothers that nurse frequently produce more dilute (watery) milk with higher carbohydrate and lower protein percentages. Humans are among these mammals.

3. A baby's sleep is different from a child's or an adult's sleep because it is the baby's job to keep you near by.

Babies instinctively know they should be with their mothers constantly. Why? Our bodies, brains, hormones, and instincts are designed to optimize survival in a hunter–gather world. Until a child is old enough to run away from danger on her own, that child is fully dependent on having its primary adult nearby.

Babies are doing their jobs when they wake frequently. They sleep differently as babies than they will later as children, teenagers, or adults. Babies have shorter sleep cycles and spend less sleep time in deep sleep. This means they can wake more easily and notice when they are no longer in physical contact with another human being.

It is not your imagination your baby wakes up almost every time you put him down, out of your arms, onto a bed. To feel safe and, thus, able to sleep, the baby depends on physical cues: feeling your heartbeat, your body warmth, your nipple in her mouth, and the sensation of rhythmic rocking from being carried on your body.

Many of us retain these sleep cues as adults. You may find that you sleep more soundly or more easily in a car, on a train, or on a plane. The rhythmic movement along with the soothing white noise that sometimes mimics a heartbeat, especially in a car, encourages a deep sleep for many people.

Ariana, a mother of twins in Ithaca, New York, told me that her babies would sleep for hours in a sling, but would never nap for more than fifteen minutes in the bassinette. Rather than fight Nature, Ariana worked with it. Her innovative solution was to add weight lifting to her life so that carrying two babies through naps was easier on her body.

You might find your baby is more sensitive to one or more of the physical sleep cues than the others. Think of all the things parents use to try to help a baby go to sleep: a white noise machine, the sound of running water, a swing, a bouncer, the motion of a car or washing machine, a pacifier, or a finger to suck on. Although pacifiers are probably better introduced after breastfeeding is well established, the rest of these can be lifesaving tricks for new parents. Still, it's important to remember that your baby is designed to keep an adult nearby—she is just doing her job.

The One with the Sleep Problem Is YOU!

So, your baby is naturally wired to keep you nearby and to feed very frequently. Does this mean you can never feel rested again? Not necessarily! But it does often require more work and scheduling than you probably anticipated before you had a baby. If we accept the biology of our baby, we can go to work on the real problem: finding a way for YOU to get sleep.

In the old days, this was a bit easier than it is today. The secret of our foremothers was their sisters, mothers, and friends. Babies grew up with a built-in village. Anthropologists tell us that sharing baby and childcare responsibilities is a human trait that dates back a very long time, and continues today among people who live away from industrialization. In villages around the world, a mother is able to prepare food, clean, and nap while another person takes care of the baby. Babies are held, and even nursed, by other women. Anthropologists give this practice the fancy term, "allomaternal lactation." It makes sense, when you think about it, that cultures across time and space would adopt practices that make it easier for mothers to continue to get or make food, and for infants to survive. And because women around the world, even today, tend to breastfeed far longer than we do in the West—the average length of breastfeeding worldwide is 4.5 years—it is easier in these other societies to find another lactating mother with whom to share some of these responsibilities. Beyond shared lactation, just having more arms available helps new mothers cope with the added responsibility of a baby. Western culture tends to frown on all maternal lactation, but more help in other areas can still lead to more rest for you.

Solutions to Try

1. Sleep with your baby if that gets you more sleep—even if it is not your long-term plan.

Many parents plan to sleep with their newborns, but many others plan to sleep separately. Despite expectations during pregnancy, most parents end up sleeping with their baby at least a little bit. This is especially true during the deep-sleep hours of the middle of the night and the "please-let-me-sleep-a-little-longer" hours of early morning.

If you are comfortable bed-sharing or room-sharing with your infant, you already reap the sleep benefits of not having to get out of bed to deal with nighttime waking. You may still need other strategies (following), because even co-sleeping mothers do not always get enough sleep!

If you are not sleeping with your baby, let me offer you permission to do so with the understanding that your goal is, eventually, to sleep apart from your child. I tell all my doula clients, "Do not do anything today because you are afraid of a future habit."

Your baby will change every day before your eyes. "Habits" of the first weeks will change dramatically, without any effort on your part, just because your baby is growing and developing so much. Likewise, the "habits" of a baby who is three months old tell you absolutely nothing about the "habits" of that same baby at nine months or eighteen months. Babies change because they have internal drives to develop new skills.

If you read online blogs or visit chat rooms, you'll see that babies learning to crawl and walk often change their sleeping patterns at the same time. Do not be afraid, in these early months, that you will develop a sleeping habit in your child you cannot change. You can always make changes when *you* are ready—which might be when you are more rested and healed.

People tend to think about sleeping with their baby as an all-or-nothing decision, when, in fact, for most people, it is a constantly evolving process. Many parents who have a strong preference for the baby sleeping in a different room end up sleeping with their baby because it helps them get more sleep in the first weeks and months. Kathleen Kendall-Tackett, a leading researcher into mother–infant sleep, points out that the cultural and medical-world message that babies should sleep in cribs on their backs leads to a rise in unsafe sleeping practices.

Ironically, this is exactly the problem this message was aimed at curing. Sleep-deprived women get out of their beds at night, walk down the hallway, and sit up in a chair or on a couch to breastfeed their baby, and

Safe Sleeping Practices

1. Breastfeed your baby.

2. Don't smoke. If quitting smoking is challenging, get help in any way you can.

3. Do not sleep with your baby if you have been drinking alcohol or have used any kind of drug (including medications) that affect your level of awareness or drowsiness. Medicines for colds, allergies, and coughs can make you less likely to wake up if your baby is moving or making sounds.

4. Do not put your baby to sleep on a couch or sleep with your baby on a couch. The same is true of waterbeds and futons that are not firm or have a wavy surface.

5. Use tight-fitting sheets on the mattress.

6. Do not allow your baby to sleep with a pillow or other objects, such as a stuffed animal.

7. Use warm clothing for your baby instead of a blanket. Mothers can get creative about their blankets (just on your legs, perhaps) or sleeping attire. I bought a zip-up fleece gown that kept me as warm as a blanket.

8. Put your baby to sleep on his back. Breastfeeding mothers in bed naturally do this most of the time.

9. Do not allow babies to sleep in beds with pets.

You have a lot of control over the most important risk factors. The first four items on the list above are so influential that if you just did those four things *and* your baby was born after thirty-seven weeks, you reduce the risk of SIDS to a negligible amount.

It's useful to know your baby is roughly 25 percent less likely to be affected by SIDS if she was born at term. Babies born before thirty-seven weeks are more at risk.

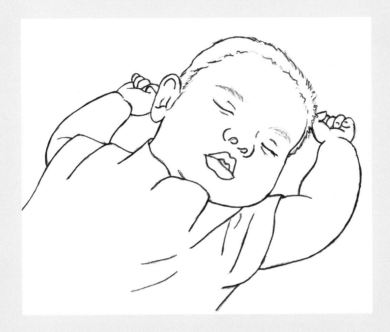

It's also helpful to know a few things about the American Academy of Pediatricians (AAP) sleep recommendations, which are a little different than those presented here. The AAP wanted to make simple and universal recommendations to new parents. The evidence about SIDS and bed-sharing is complicated by the fact that researchers do not distinguish between bed-sharing in a bed with a firm mattress and bed-sharing on couches, chairs, waterbeds, or futons. Rather than parse this to the public, the AAP decided to recommend against *all* bed-sharing, even though the evidence does not warrant this.

Based on research by Kathleen Kendall-Tackett, Ph.D.
For more information, visit her website at
www.uppitysciencechick.com/KKTtearsheet_FINALrevised.pdf

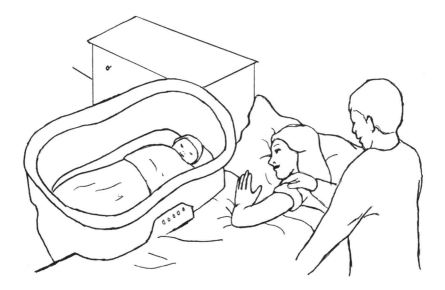

often fall asleep there. Sleeping with your baby on a couch is far more dangerous than sleeping with your baby in your bed!

Be flexible when you think about where your baby sleeps. There are more options than you might, at first, realize. Maybe you put your baby down in a crib for the first long sleep of the night and then take him into your bed for the rest of the night. Maybe you co-sleep with your baby in your bed, but later end up sleeping in another room because you can sleep with less distraction there.

A mattress on the floor is a solution many mothers advocate. Chelsea, from Santa Cruz, California, explained she would breastfeed her baby to sleep in the evening on a twin mattress on the floor. Then, about an hour or two later, she was able to go to bed with her husband in their regular bed. In the middle of the night, she climbed down to the baby's twin mattress on the floor to breastfeed. Sometimes, she stayed there until morning. Sometimes, if she had to go the bathroom, she'd get back in the big bed. Chelsea notes, "This worked better for me than a co-sleeper, because I could move my baby from side to side to breastfeed without waking up my husband and I could stretch out fully and sleep while my baby was eating." Other mothers put a daybed in the baby's room for the same purpose. This "best of both worlds" approach allows you to co-sleep and have your own marital bed at the same time.

Finally, if you planned to co-sleep but discover your baby is happier sleeping apart from you, it is fine to deviate from the plan you developed during pregnancy. This happens less often than the reverse, but it does happen. Respecting your unique baby's needs is a sign you are a caring parent.

2. Ask other adults to watch your baby so you can sleep.

If you have relatives or friends who have offered to help, this is a concrete, wonderful way they can do so. In the first six months —and even after, if needed—I hope you will throw away societal norms and embrace a "receiver's heart." Instead of feeling like you are putting your relatives or friends out by asking for babysitting in exchange for sleep, know you are giving them the gift of being able to help you in a meaningful way.

Margo, who lived in Manhattan when her first baby was born, let her mother-in-law, Janice, take her baby for a long walk in the stroller every Wednesday afternoon. In good weather, they walked outside. In bad weather, they went to museums. If she could, Margo fed her baby right before this walk, so she'd have the longest possible time for a nap. Even if that didn't work, if her baby was asleep at the time Janice arrived, Janice always took the baby away for the afternoon. Throughout the week, Margo pumped a small amount of milk that her mother-in-law fed to the baby with a dropper, if needed, because they had not started to use bottles yet. In this way, Margo was able to get a four-hour nap every Wednesday that she describes as "lifesaving." She says, "It was like I could get through all the long nights because I knew there would be this blissful, uninterrupted sleep coming my way—even if it were days away! I lived for Wednesday afternoons!"

I asked how her mother-in-law handled the baby crying, and Margo said, "I don't think he cried too much for her. I just kept telling myself that she loves him and, even if he's crying, he's with someone who loves him."

You may not have a mother-in-law who can implement such a routine plan. But if you start off asking for help at least one afternoon or morning a week, it can be rejuvenating enough to help you get through the hard moments. A mother in my town who lived far from all family was willing to ask neighbors and acquaintances for help. She found this became a way to build deeper friendships. She advises, "Be vulnerable! Ask for help. You will be happy to return the favor someday."

I highly recommend that you ask well-meaning relatives and friends to contribute toward the cost of a postpartum doula in lieu of baby gifts.

If you live far away from family and are new enough in town not to have friendships to lean on for such help, hire a postpartum doula for this purpose. In addition to being able to sleep when the doula comes over, you'll be able to get answers to routine questions about infant feeding or care and, possibly, some laundry and dishes done. Although more expensive than a minimum-wage babysitter, postpartum doulas have training and experience with newborns and new mothers.

3. Sleep whenever it is possible—day or night!

Consider every hour in your twenty-four-hour day as potential sleep time. An unconscious barrier for many new mothers is the Western idea that adult sleep must happen within the rigid parameters of 10 p.m. to 7 a.m. Sleeping at 2 p.m. is considered a "nap." But for the first six weeks of your baby's life, you will get the most sleep if you follow the age-old advice to "sleep when your baby sleeps."

Although you will likely hear this from several sources, I extend this advice to include, "And also sleep when your baby is awake and happy and someone else can play with her!" Of course, you want to play with your baby during her awake and alert stages. There will be other awake and alert moments, and you will enjoy them *more* if you are rested.

Your hormones and your body will adjust to the frequent waking and intermittent sleeping pattern better than you might imagine—and certainly better than a nonlactating person would adapt to such a schedule. Your new hormones support this kind of sleep. Your body is making milk, filling your breasts, and making you feel the best if you are able to breastfeed frequently. When you feed your baby, you release "sleepy" hormones, so even during the day you might find yourself nodding off during or after a feeding. Take advantage of this instead of fighting it. If you were someone who had trouble getting to or staying asleep, throw away your ideas about yourself. This is a new world! You will be getting sleep cues in new and different ways.

The Initial "Long-ish" Sleep and How to Use It

At around four to six weeks, most mothers can distinguish a longer sleep period that seems like the "beginning of the night" for the baby. This is the sleep period in which your baby is most likely to stay asleep, in a bed or bassinette, without constant physical contact. After the first stretch of sleep, some babies have a second long stretch (another three or four hours in a row) and some babies start waking up more often (every hour or every two hours or so). Another common experience is that babies will wake up and be alert in the morning for about two hours—and then fall into another exhausted, long nap in the early morning.

The longer, initial night sleep can begin virtually any time between 6 p.m. and 2 a.m., but it will usually be somewhat predictable. After being the mother to one night owl and then an early bird, I was not surprised to learn that research suggests whichever one you are is a hard-wired characteristic. This preference is called "chronotype," and it is hard to change in any individual—including your infant! That said, babies do often take about six weeks to adjust to life in a world with sunshine and nighttime, so don't despair right away if you and your baby don't seem to share a fondness for early mornings or late evenings. Around six weeks or so, most babies adjust to the twenty-four-hour cycle and their chronotypes become obvious.

Whether your baby is asleep at 6:30 p.m. or 1:30 a.m., I urge you to make a conscious choice about what to do with this first chunk of nighttime sleep. This is your best chance to get your own "deep sleep" (non-REM slow-wave sleep) and get through two cycles of it in a row before you are woken up. This is *also* your best chance to do anything that you can't do with a wakeful infant, or one who won't stay asleep unless she's in your arms. This is when you want to eat a delicious meal, talk to your spouse, return your best friend's phone call, and take a shower. It won't be long before you also consider using this time to explore your sexual self with your partner again. (See chapter 6, page 163.) But making a habit of staying awake to be an adult can lead to exhaustion.

My personal advice is:

- Do anything you can do with the baby, *with* the baby (for example, taking a bath is a great activity to do with a baby).
- Don't use evening sleep time for any chores.
- Always prioritize sleep in the first six weeks.

This may be impractical to implement every day, because you do need to nurture yourself, so consider a 2:1 plan. Two nights, you go to sleep with your baby for the long, initial sleep and one night you are an adult during that time. The important thing is that baby's first long night sleep is time for you to refresh—so whatever you do during that time should have that effect. Doing chores and paying bills is draining. Use a morning or afternoon to do those. Sleep or otherwise renew yourself while your baby sleeps.

Special Circumstances

Some new mothers go into the postpartum period already aware they have trouble sleeping. Others develop insomnia after giving birth. In any case, it is one of the cruelest ironies to deprive new mothers of any sleep at all for any reason besides a baby's needs. In your case, you may need more rhythm and predictability, which will probably require even more help from your partner, relatives, or friends to make this a reality. Your baby is unlikely to help you get to bed at the same time every evening, but your partner can certainly try.

Insomnia

Winona, a mother of four boys in western Montana, shares her experience living with insomnia, which she clearly refined over the years of having several children. I always love such advice because first-time moms can learn from the experience, too, without having to have four children first.

> I remember being so desperate as postpartum insomnia had me in its clutches. The baby would sleep, but I would lie there. I went to the health food store, and melatonin was the only option they offered me. I was hesitant to use it as a couple family members had bad side effects from it. I ended up finding a routine that did really help.

> "I would put the baby in the swing or in the bouncer (and bounce it with my foot). Usually that got the baby to sleep pretty easily and I could start my routine.

> "I would make sure to have calcium and magnesium supplements at bedtime. I used a liquid supplement from a natural company that worked well. I would read on the couch, all ready for bed. First I would have a high-protein, low-carb snack with chamomile tea. Then I'd brush my teeth and read for a while. When I absolutely could not keep my eyes open, I would go straight to bed, turn out the lights, and generally fall asleep. However, I discovered, too, that sometimes it was my brain that kept me awake. So, finding something that would occupy my brain, but that I was familiar with, like a familiar TV show with the monitor turned off or audio book, would do the trick and I would be asleep like I took a sleeping pill.

Apps for Insomnia

If you are having trouble getting to sleep yourself, listening to a CD or online recording can be just the thing you need to relax and fall asleep. As my friend Lakshmi says, "I often toss and turn in bed and forget that I have options."

- "Relax and Refocus" is an MP3 or CD from Jennifer Elliot at lifesjourney.ca/hypnosis-recordings/#relax
- "Deep Sleep with Andrew Johnson" by Michael Schneider is a guided meditation available through iTunes.
- Insight Timer is a meditation app available at https://insighttimer.com
- Headspace meditation guides are available through headspace.com

Insomnia is an awful burden, but you probably know it responds best to routines of waking and going to bed at the same time, getting adequate exercise, and calming therapies such as mindfulness meditation. If you have not tried these before, you can start:

- **A routine:** As Winona relates previously, a going-to-bed ritual can help your body understand it is time to wind down and go to sleep. Experts advise going to bed and waking up at the same time every day, which is not, at all, easy with a newborn.

- **Avoiding stimulants:** It's important not to use caffeine to stay awake during the day, as tempting as it is.

- **Exercise:** A good walk every day, after the first two to four weeks, is more important for mothers with insomnia than anyone else. It helps release tension and gets you into natural sunlight, which helps your body understand when to be awake and when to sleep.

- **A plan to reduce worrying:** Mindfulness meditation or another stress-reducing therapy can help quiet your mind. If you've never tried mindfulness meditation, this is the time to do it! Progressive muscle relaxation is a wonderful strategy that only takes a few minutes, and that you can do in bed next to a newborn. There is a multitude of wonderful phone apps these days for meditation and muscle relaxation that help you get to sleep.

Your Baby Never Sleeps More Than Thirty- to Sixty-Minute Stretches, Even at Night, or Your Baby Is Extremely Colicky

Oh, Mama! The rest of us feel for you. This is so hard and there is little anyone can say to make it feel any easier on you.

A difficult fact of life is that you, the mother, have to acknowledge that if your baby is extremely colicky, or for any other reason sleeps poorly, you are going through something arduous. Ask for help, even if it is not your nature to do so. Everyone knows the newborn period is difficult, but if your baby won't allow you to complete a sleep cycle, your situation is harder than average. Like parents whose babies are in the NICU, you deserve special support.

You will probably just have to survive the first six weeks any way you can. Though this is a stressful situation, take heart that experienced mothers say things do get better, often around the six-week mark and, again, at around three months. Lean on your partner, your relatives, and your friends more than you would normally. If your baby is not giving you three or four hours of sleep in a row, you must have help. It is not sustainable. If you have trouble asking for help, know that you must. It's not an option to soldier through this. Adults cannot function with so many sleep interruptions.

Any new mother without relatives or close friends who can offer reliable baby help should consider hiring a postpartum doula. But, in your case, I wish I could convince physicians and midwives to prescribe a postpartum doula as a health necessity. In some countries, postpartum nurses *do* come to your home to help for free. Those government officials realize there is a long-term benefit to making sure all mothers and babies do well in the first months. If you absolutely cannot afford a postpartum doula (but let me urge you to look in every budget category to find the money to do this!), get creative about finding help. Even a thirteen-year-old mother's helper, who plays with your baby while you take a nap, is better than nothing.

Mothers whose infants are so wakeful or colicky should also enlist help for cooking meals and cleaning more than other mothers. First-time mothers often have a harder time making this a reality because they are not connected to other parents through an older child. I found that the parents of my older children's playmates and classmates were the most likely to bring us food when I had my second and third child. Read, "Planning a Meal Train" (page 37), even if you are six- or twelve-weeks postpartum already. It's never too late.

Determine Whether Your Baby Has GERD Get professional help to rule out physical causes of your baby's wakefulness or crankiness. Not sleeping more than thirty- to sixty-minute bouts is a common symptom of gastroesophageal reflux disease (GERD), also called acid reflux. So is extreme fussiness. It will usually take a few weeks to establish that the problem is due to acid reflux and is not just normal newborn adjustment to life outside the womb. If this sleep or crying pattern continues past about four weeks and is accompanied by any other GERD symptoms, it is definitely worth an evaluation. Other symptoms include spitting up more than usual (this may be hard for first-time parents to determine on their own); fussiness that increases when the baby is in a lying-down position; choking or gagging during feeding; and/or crying during a feeding or right after a feeding (most babies are calmed by feeding). GERD in infants is usually worse until around four months, at which time it often starts to get better, and most babies grow out of GERD by their first birthday. But you need help before that, so please consult your midwife or pediatrician.

Try Probiotics Infant gut and digestion problems may indicate baby's gut was not colonized properly at birth. You should suspect this especially if you or your baby received antibiotics during late pregnancy, labor, or postpartum, or if you had a cesarean. Babies normally receive their first dose of bacteria to colonize their gut when being born through the vaginal canal. So, if your baby was not exposed to your vaginal bacteria at all (as in a cesarean), or a dose of antibiotics killed off these bacteria, he may need external probiotics to help him digest his food. This was not well understood a generation ago, but gut bacteria are the subject of increasing numbers of scientific studies. More and more health issues are being connected to the health of our guts.

Health food stores generally carry probiotics designed specifically for infants. If you do not live near such a store, these are easy to purchase online. Usually, they come in powder form that you refrigerate. When you give the probiotics to your baby, simply mix the powder into your breastmilk and feed your baby with a small medicine cup. You can sit him up on your lap with your hand behind his neck. Tip his head back a little bit and dribble the liquid into his mouth. I recommend brands that do not contain dairy, because dairy is such a common allergen.

Try an Elimination Diet If GERD is an issue (or suspected issue) for a breastfed baby, you might try an elimination diet, too, to see if your baby is experiencing pain because of an allergen in your breastmilk. Dairy is the allergen scientific research has been able to link most successfully with infant colic. Try to eliminate dairy products from your own diet for three weeks (four would be even better). Keep track of whether there is improvement in sleep or fussiness. It's important to know that lactose-free products will not work for an elimination diet because the problem is often the dairy protein, not the lactose sugar.

If dairy is not the culprit, try other possible allergens. If there is any history of allergy in your families, use that history as a guide. A good place to start, if you'd like to learn more about elimination diets and food sensitivities, is: http://kellymom.com/health/baby-health/food-sensitivity.

A caution about elimination diets: I see many mothers who eliminate potential allergens in their diet to help their babies. I support women in experimenting to find what works for them. However, I see a lot of mothers who *stay* on restricted diets because their babies are fussy or wakeful, but who do not ever know for certain that their diet helps. I suspect they feel they must do everything they can—and diet is an area over which they have control. But there is no need to be on a gluten-free, dairy-free, soy-free, sugar-free diet as a breastfeeding mother UNLESS it actually makes your life better. So, if you try an elimination diet and it does not improve your life, please do not stay on it.

Determine Whether Musculoskeletal Pain Is an Issue Many mothers with colicky and wakeful babies suspect their baby is in pain, but cannot pinpoint it exactly. Chiropractors suggest something in the musculoskeletal system might have been moved out of place during the baby's birth. If something is not quite right at the musculoskeletal level, your baby may be in pain when you hold her in certain positions to eat or when she lies down to sleep. Many parents try avenues such as chiropractic care, craniosacral therapy, Reiki, and infant massage. Roxanne, who runs "The Holistic Mama" website, had four fussy babies with acid reflux. She found that chiropractic care helped her third child and told me:

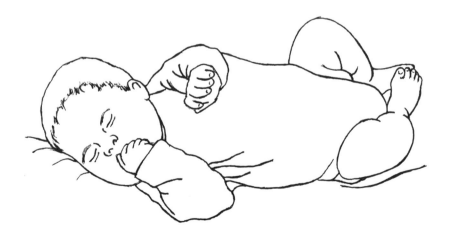

This one was the winner for my third baby. He screamed inces-santly for the first nine weeks of his life. Every other thing we tried helped a little, but he was still miserable. When he was two months old, we moved and I was able to try a different chiropractor, and the results were instant and lasting. He stopped screaming during the adjustment, fell asleep, and slept for nine hours straight (he'd slept only twenty to thirty minutes at a time up until that point!) When he woke the next day he was happy and content.

Most therapies for musculoskeletal pain come with a relatively high initial cost, although return visits are usually less expensive. Infant massage is a low-cost, do-it-yourself option you might enjoy even if it does not magically fix your baby's sleep or fussiness problem. Videos on infant massage abound, so you can learn this helpful skill easily. In some communities there are classes, which I highly recommend, because watching a skilled baby masseuse gives you lots of ideas and allows you to meet other new parents.

Conclusion

By now, you know I think your baby is probably getting enough sleep (unless she has GERD or pain), but that you, probably, are not. This is not the same advice you will receive in most baby sleep books—or in online chat rooms about infant sleep. I've seen new parents reeling with anger and frustration because they can't get their infant to sleep even after following expert suggestions closely. I find this reframing useful: If parents focus their efforts on getting sleep themselves, much frustra-tion can be avoided. This frustrating period of no sleep will end. It will get better. I know it does not help you in the moment, but all of us who have been through it know that, eventually, you will sleep again and we are rooting for you.

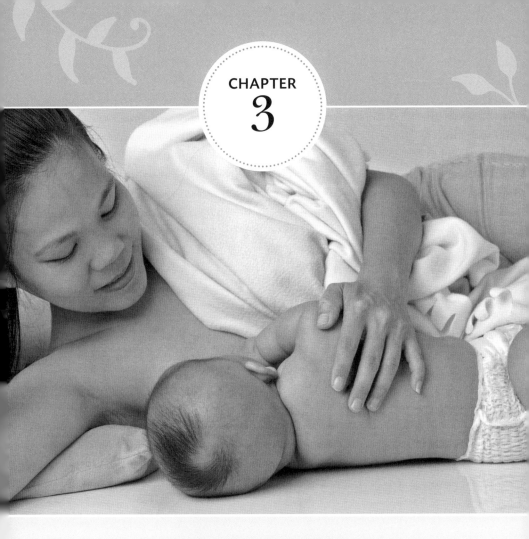

SELF-CARE, INFANT CARE, AND INFANT FEEDING

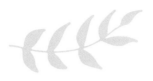

A CHAPTER ON INFANT CARE SHOULD START WITH the parent's self-care. This is the truth about our children: They are insatiable! I don't mean simply physically insatiable, although two hours into a nursing marathon can feel that way. I mean they have insatiable needs and desires that could take up all our waking hours, if we let them. If you start from this premise, you are more likely to understand the necessity of making time for self-care. You can never wait until your baby (or older child) is completely settled to begin taking care of yourself. If that were the case, you would be holding your breath for eighteen years.

Instead, find the sweet spot that D. W. Winnicott has called "good enough parenting." Good enough parenting acknowledges that parents have needs and wants, too, and the family functions best when parents are able to take care of themselves *and* their children. Maintaining control over our own mindless and, frankly, addictive behavior around technology can help us become better people and better parents. We begin our "infant-care" discussion with a look at parenting that works for both parents and children.

There are also some basic things you should know about infant care that may not be obvious to first-time parents. For example, when I see new parents at the first postpartum visit, they are usually concerned about sleep, baby's first bath, cord care, diapering, and infant feeding. Sleep is such a big issue for parents that I tackle it in its own chapter (chapter 2, page 47). Here, I discuss other major concerns from smallest to largest. The second half of the chapter is devoted to infant feeding.

Infant Care

Let's reflect, for a moment, on what we intend to do as parents. If you have a journal for yourself, or are keeping a baby book, this is a beautiful exercise to complete. Simply ask yourself what your parenting goals are, now that this sweet being is in your care.

First put on your own oxygen mask—modeling self-care is part of parenting.

As I understand it, the main goal of parenting is to nurture children in a way that encourages them to grow up to be three things: as autonomous as their ability and potential allow; ethical and kind in their interactions with themselves and others (which includes having a positive self-image); able to learn and grow in understanding, skill-development, and creativity throughout their entire lives. In reality, these goals must bend to fit who we are, and who our children are. A child with disabilities may have a different level of potential autonomy than another child, for example.

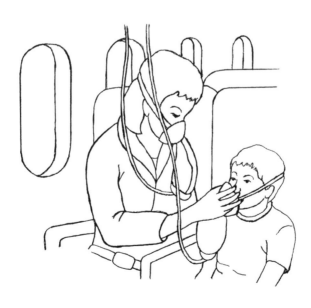

So, how do we help our children attain these lofty goals? One part of the answer is being attentive to our children, and meeting their emotional, physical, intellectual, and spiritual needs. This is the basis of attachment parenting: Children learn to trust that the world is safe and good, and that they, themselves, are good, because of the way their parents met their needs as infants and children. Victor Bloom, M.D., explains how it works: "Self-esteem comes from the internal representation (memory) of a good (loving) parent." However, if we focus solely on meeting our children's needs, we will burn out, because, as I've noted already, children are insatiable.

Another part of the answer—often forgotten—is that we must also model how to be a good, kind, loving person *to one's self.* Being self-sacrificing to the point of exhausting yourself is clearly unhealthy and unsustainable. What surprises some parents, who are desperately trying to entertain and enrich their baby's life for optimum development, is that this martyrdom philosophy is also unhealthy for the child.

One of my favorite books on childcare is *You Are Your Child's First Teacher,* by Rahima Baldwin Dancy. This book is based on the philosophy of Rudolf Steiner, a mystic who lived about a century ago. One of Steiner's insights is that children learn in different ways at different ages. From birth to age seven, children learn by imitation. Dancy points out that parents and teachers need to cultivate their own lives to offer effective nurturance to children. We expect teachers everywhere to engage in "professional development," but this often means taking classes on effective teaching methods. Teachers who follow Steiner's philosophy are supposed to work on their own artistic, intellectual, and spiritual development. Because children learn through imitation, they develop more fully when their parents and teachers grow as well.

You must be living a life that can be imitated. If you are only engaged in child care, there is nothing for your child to emulate. Doing the dishes near your child is not ignoring her, it is teaching her.

Part of modeling how to be a good, kind, capable human is modeling how to handle your mistakes. "Here's the thing. You're going to mess this parenting thing up. The sooner you accept it, the sooner you can stop being so worried about messing this parenting thing up," Dawn Dais wrote in her tongue-in-cheek book, *The Sh!t No One Tells You: A Guide to Surviving Your Baby's First Year*, (page 191). New parents bring home these tiny, precious babes, and often spend the first weeks of this precious fourth trimester on tenterhooks, afraid to make a mistake. But you absolutely will make mistakes! Throwing away any ideas you have about not doing so will serve you well for many years to come. Being willing to admit your mistakes and make amends is how your children learn to take risks, fail, and learn from their own mistakes. Although we worry our mistakes will harm our children, it's helpful to remember that while children are insatiable, they are also resilient.

Regulate the Level of Stimulation for You and Your Baby

One of the first and biggest mistakes new parents make is believing their child needs constant stimulation. This leads to frantic attempts to play the right music, introduce colors and patterns at optimal times, and speak the correct number of words to their infant per day. Parents feel guilty for not doing enough, or for talking on the phone with a sister or friend instead of "stimulating" junior.

Your baby loves to be near you and, in the first weeks, loves to touch you. Satisfying this need is a priority. However, your baby comes with an inborn drive to learn, and is learning all the time. At first, he is simply learning about his own body and how to make his arms and legs and head move voluntarily. Yes, his eyes are learning how to discern shapes and patterns, but there are shapes and patterns virtually everywhere. Your baby does not need special exposure to these.

Dancy describes two factors that contribute to our modern-day guilt and exhaustion as parents. First, we often parent in isolation, far away from extended family members. She describes the experience of a friend living in rural Mexico at the time, and practicing attachment parenting, wearing her baby most of the time. As the child grew, this mother came to realize she was more exhausted than her Mexican counterparts. She had assumed that she, alone, should provide all, or most, of that baby-wearing care, while the Mexican women shared this responsibility with extended family.

Secondly, Dancy points out that many of us tend to "focus on the child instead of on the work of homemaking" we could be doing while at home with a baby. This is not good for either parent or child, she claims, because, "Modern life simply doesn't support what young children need, which is to see us doing work that involves movement or . . . transformation of materials—something they can both share in and then imitate in their play." You know well enough you don't get the same sense of satisfaction from noodling around on Facebook that you do from real-world work, such as finishing a project, planting seeds in a garden, or even getting the dishes done before bed.

Although infants are not yet ready to share in or mimic our daily work, it is the rhythms of life we are imparting now. Previously this was

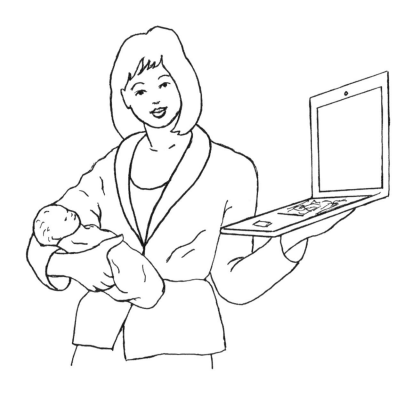

done effortlessly. Today it takes a more conscious effort to get off the phone and computer, to sweep a floor instead of sending a remote vacuum across the house, and to wash, chop, and sauté vegetables instead of ordering take-out. Certainly, the judicious use of technology can improve our lives. For example, during the winter in New York City, where I lived without a car, online grocery ordering was a godsend. Still, what your baby may need most from you—and what you may need for yourself—is conscious limitations on the technology that ceaselessly beckons us.

Once you get the hang of nursing, you may find yourself mindlessly swiping through social media on your phone. There may be nothing wrong with this, per se, but I have personally experienced a calmer, more relaxed nursing time when I chose to focus my attention on the baby and myself. If I sat still for a moment, I could feel where my body was aching and needed a good stretch. I am not good at controlling my impulses on my phone, and I would soon be answering texts or emails. I intentionally make rules for myself regarding when and where I want to answer texts and emails, and when I will spend time on social media. One of my clients made it a practice to spend the first two or three minutes of each nursing simply being present with her baby. Then she would either read a book, if she were sitting up, or listen to a podcast, if she were lying down.

Online groups can be an invaluable tool to find answers to questions quickly. While I was writing this book, I posed many parenting questions to online groups and usually got dozens of answers in less than a day. I encourage you to use these groups for the support they can offer, but also make it a habit to connect with like-minded people in the world around you. In-person groups have even more to offer than their online counterparts. (There is a list of possible groups to try on pages 180–181). Remember that your baby, and eventually your older child, will learn how to relate to other people by *watching and imitating you* She, literally, cannot learn the rhythm of a conversation through typing. Your children need to see you exploring human interactions across a variety of contexts.

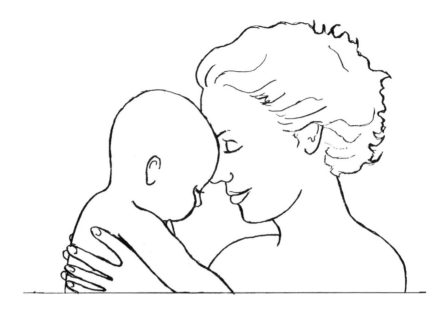

Newborn Care

Bathing Your Baby

If you give birth in a hospital, you can request that the nurses not bathe your baby. At the teaching hospital near me, this is becoming more and more common. In the first day or two of life, if you've declined a bath for your baby, you may want to rub the vernix coating into the baby's skin and simply wet-towel off any blood or other fluids, especially from the hair. Then, if you want to wait a few days to a week for a full bath, that is absolutely fine.

Babies are not actually "dirty" and they have no way to accumulate dirt in their first weeks of life, so they do not require much bathing for cleanliness. You likely clean her private area several times a day as you diaper, anyway. Some parents love giving their baby a bath in a special tub, or in the kitchen sink, as part of a bedtime routine. Partners are especially good at handling this often-lovely experience.

If your baby appears to hate baths, do keep trying. Babies change fast and what leads to crying one day could be calming the next. Your baby might have fussed because they feel too open, floppy, and exposed in a baby tub. They might prefer to be held in a bathtub or wrapped in a towel. You can just keep the towel around the baby as you put them in the tub.

Consider taking baths *with* your baby—but for relaxation or routine—not because your baby needs a bath. Some care providers still recommend waiting to take a bath until your stitches or incisions are healed, but most agree that herbal baths are healing for mom and baby. You can brew special herbs on your stove and always have a pot ready to pour into your bath. You can purchase premade herb mixtures (from Earth Mama Angel Baby, Birth Song Botanicals, or Herb Lore, for example), or mix them yourself.

Garlic is a wonderful ingredient for these baths—it is naturally antibacterial and antiviral. Uva ursi leaves and comfrey are also antimicrobial. These three ingredients are beneficial to any open wounds on you and your baby. Plantain has properties that speed healing by spurring the growth of new cells. Together, these herbs help your perineum and/or your cesarean incision areas heal, and also promote good health for your baby's cord. A simple recipe is included in this chapter (see page 78).

Cord Care

Older advice recommends cleaning umbilical cords using rubbing alcohol on a cotton swab, and keeping it completely dry until it falls off. Today, most doctors and midwives say the best thing to do is absolutely nothing. The cord will dry out and fall off on its own without your help. Submerging the cord area in water is fine and, in the case of an herbal bath, probably even helpful. Just make sure the area is completely dry after the bath. Submersion in water actually causes the cord to dry out more quickly than it would otherwise. You can leave it exposed to air until it dries or use a cotton swab.

DIY Postpartum Herbal Bath for Mamas and Babies

Use what you have. If you are missing an ingredient, it's not a big deal. Order some of these online, as herbal teas, if they are hard to find in your town. Good places to find herbs include your local co-op, a local herbalist, Mountain Rose Herbs, Starwest Botanicals, or Amazon.

In addition to the following ingredients, other nice additions include dried lavender or red raspberry leaf tea.

- ½ to 1 cup (60 g to 120 g) colloidal oatmeal (see Note)
- ½ cup (32 g) dried calendula flowers, or 4 to 5 chamomile tea bags
- ¼ to ½ cup (62.5 g to 125 g) Epsom salt, or (72 g to 144 g) sea salt
- ¼ cup (32 g) dried uva ursi leaf
- ¼ cup (10 g) dried plantain leaf
- 1 or 2 cloves of garlic

1. In a large pot over high heat, combine the oatmeal, calendula flowers, Epsom salt, uva ursi leaf, plantain, and garlic with 2 gallons (7.5 L) water and bring to a boil. Turn the heat to low and simmer for 1 to 2 hours. Let the mixture sit in the pot overnight. If you are not brewing ahead of time, reduce the simmering time to 20 minutes and use it right away. You can use this mixture while it is hot (mixed into bath water) or let it cool.

2. Pour the mixture through a strainer or cloth into the bath. You can also add this mixture to your peri bottle to wash your perineum after using the bathroom. If you make extra, keep it refrigerated in a covered container for up to one week.

Note: *If you don't have colloidal oatmeal, use any kind of oatmeal you have, even instant. These flakes will be larger, though, so blend these oatmeals into finer pieces for the bath. A clean coffee grinder or blender will do the trick.*

For more ideas, look online for recipes and explanations about herbs by Demetria Clark, director of Heart of Herbs Herbal School, and Birth Arts International. Aviva Romm is also a popular herbalist and author with available online resources.

Of course, if you notice signs of infection, such as red streaks on the skin near the cord, pus, a terrible smell, active bleeding, or a fever, contact your care provider.

Diapering

Diapering goes hand-in-hand with infant feeding, because it is one of two signs your baby is getting enough nutrition. The other sign of adequate nutrition is your baby's weight, which you might only measure occasionally if feeding is going well. Nonetheless, wet and dirty diapers are a daily record of your baby's health.

It's a good idea to keep track of the wet and dirty diapers during the first week, when most babies have lost a little weight after birth and are just beginning to gain, until you are sure your baby is gaining steadily. For many babies, this could be as early as the second week.

Prior to your milk coming in, normal output is considered at least one wet and one dirty diaper per day. After your milk has come in, the normal minimum amount increases to six wet diapers and three to four stool diapers per day. Some babies will pee and poo even more.

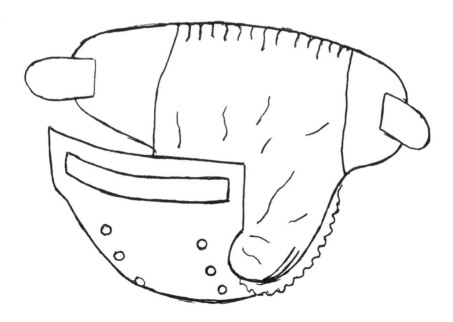

If you are concerned about quantity, gauge them this way: Stools should be about the size of a quarter (although some babies are capable of releasing quite a bit more) and the urine should be at least a tablespoon (15 ml). Babies have tiny bladders, so they need to empty them frequently. Baby's pee should be almost colorless, although it is helpful for new parents to know that some babies may have pinkish urine in the first days. This is normal and will pass. The color of your baby's stools will change after the first day or two, when it is dark, blackish, and called "meconium." If you breastfeed your baby, the stool will get lighter in color over the course of a few days until it is a mustardy-yellow shade. The consistency of a breastfed baby's poo resembles cottage cheese. Formula-fed babies will have more peanut-buttery poo that is on the brown spectrum.

After about the first week, you can relax about keeping such close records. However, you may continue to notice and discuss your baby's output for weeks, or even months, in ways you could not have imagined before having children of your own.

After about three weeks, some babies continue to poop several times a day, while others slow down dramatically. At my mother–baby group, it was common for a mother to arrive slightly panicked about her baby having not pooped for days. This is perfectly normal and, while you may want to consult your pediatrician for reassurance, it usually resolves itself, and might even become your baby's new pattern.

Diapers, Diapers, Diapers Natural-leaning parents often decide to use cloth diapers, or eco-friendly disposable diapers, or even a mix. I am envious of all the cloth choices available today. When I had my first baby, there were basically only large, white, flat diapers, which needed to be folded and pinned. That was it. These days, you can purchase any color in all kinds of styles.

Cloth diapering is a commitment of time and energy, but it yields great dividends for the planet, your wallet, and your baby's health. I urge you to consider investigating options. If you wash your own cloth diapers, the cost over time is significantly less than if you purchase disposable diapers. Many medium-size cities have at least one store with a variety of diaper choices and expert staff to explain the options. Visit one while you are pregnant, bring your partner or a friend, and make a date of exploring this consumer's paradise.

There are diaper services that will do all the hard work for you. All you have to do is change your baby's diaper and deposit the wet or dirty diaper in a bin that is picked up weekly. You'll get a stack of freshly laundered diapers in exchange for your stinky ones. The cost is more comparable to using disposables; however, it's a pretty great deal if you are willing to pay for it.

If you plan to launder your own diapers, plan to do a load at least every two to three days. The more similar to disposables the cloth diapers are, the more expensive they tend to be. Invest in at least two waterproof, zippered bags (or "wet bags") for soiled diapers. When you are away from home, you can easily change diapers and zip away the dirty ones. If you have a top-loading washing machine, unzipping the bag and dumping the diapers into the washer is simple enough. A front-loading machine requires slightly more arm gymnastics, but is still doable.

Cloth diapering does not have to be an all-or-nothing decision. Many parents are able to cloth diaper during the day, but choose to switch to disposables at night or when they travel. Some parents find cloth easier to handle before babies start to walk—and diaper changes often become stand-up affairs.

Elimination Communication If you are interested in being even more ecologically friendly, you can skip diapering completely by using the elimination communication (EC) method. If you pay close attention, your baby will give you physical signs he is about to pee or poop. With this method, you learn to recognize these signals and hold the baby over the toilet at the proper time. *Voilà*! No diapers needed. This method works best if a primary parent is home long-term with the infant to become wholly tuned in to the baby's cues. This is how many people around the world handle the toileting needs of babies, and it is becoming increasingly popular in the United States and Canada. If you'd like to learn more about this method, go to Diaperfreebaby. org. It provides free information and a link to find free groups that meet across the United States.

> *Starting from a humble place: Let's support all new mothers.*

Infant Feeding

I was once a smug natural-birth and parenting advocate. I have been humbled by my experiences, by my children, and by the process of interacting with thousands of new mothers and babies since I began studying reproduction in the 1990s. I once believed, for example, that most cesareans were unnecessary, and women could choose to be better prepared or more determined in their commitment to vaginal birth to avoid them. This is, indeed, true, sometimes. But now I have humbly served women who were the most prepared and committed, and whose situation still required surgical intervention. I have learned how painful it is when others judge or question their decisions.

Likewise with infant feeding, there are many more factors involved than are immediately apparent to an outsider. Some mothers desperately want to breastfeed their infants, but because of circumstances beyond their control, they find they cannot. Some women go through unspeakable pain, endless hours of pumping, or frequent medical appointments trying to provide the irreplaceable nutrition of breastmilk to their babies. Other mothers, perhaps survivors of sexual abuse or single mothers trying to hold down jobs incompatible with breastfeeding, know from the beginning that breastfeeding cannot work in their lives. All these mothers make wise, courageous choices with the resources and support they have. Some may end up bottle-feeding breastmilk (their own or donor milk), and others feed their baby formula.

There are many ways to feed your baby, and there are many ways your baby can thrive. Infant feeding can be a complex, touchy issue that, in the end, is unique to every mother–baby dyad. You may find yourself, with good reasons, anywhere on the infant-feeding spectrum: breastfeeding easily, breastfeeding with challenges, supplementing with formula, or feeding formula exclusively.

If breastmilk is available, that is the healthiest choice. The nutritional benefits of breastmilk are enormous, as are the emotional benefits to the mother and baby created by the breastfeeding relationship. But formula is a life-saving invention that I am grateful we have. I always try to assume that mothers have made the best, most thoughtful choice they could within their individual circumstances.

Breastfeeding

This section discusses how breastfeeding works in a new mother's life, without commenting much on the nitty-gritty information you might need to achieve a deeper latch, analyze how much milk your baby is consuming, or treat thrush or mastitis. More hands-on, specific information can be obtained from a postpartum doula, an IBCLC (International Board Certified Lactation Consultant), La Leche League leaders, Breastfeeding USA, WIC Peer Counselors, and online resources. Beware, though, there is a lot of bad advice online, so look for breastfeeding sites vetted by professionals. Barbara Robertson, IBCLC, offers a website (bfcaa.com) with informative podcasts, blog posts, and videos. Other sites you can trust include the International Breast-Feeding Centre (ibconline.ca) and especially Kellymom.com.

Breastfeeding Is Its Own Journey Let's begin by recognizing that breastfeeding is more of a journey than an accomplishment. Like a long hike through forest, prairie, or mountain, the terrain changes frequently. What works one day may not work well the next. There are rarely instant answers to breastfeeding challenges that will transform a difficult situation into a blissful one. There are, occasionally, tips that do feel magical, but mothers will often have to try new ideas many times before there is a shift in the right direction. Incremental progress toward your goals is much more common than bounding leaps of progress.

For some women, breastfeeding begins the hour after birth and continues without problems or issues until mother and baby are ready to wean. If this describes you, congratulations, please enjoy your breastfeeding and move on to more relevant chapters! For other mothers, however, breastfeeding has bumps and dips that require attention, care, advice, and support. In some cases, women must draw on their deepest reservoirs of strength and determination to make breastfeeding work. As lactation consultant Barbara Robertson says, "Breastfeeding can sometimes be the easiest or the hardest thing you've ever done in your life."

Good Positioning

There are many possible nursing positions, but the important thing is that you are comfortable the entire time. We have found three other factors that can help tremendously. Regardless of position, making sure the baby is well-supported, their whole body is against yours, and their chin is off their chest seem to really help. For the cradle position, the most common breastfeeding position, the baby is across your abdomen with pillow support beneath your arms. Also be conscious of leaning backward instead of hunching over your baby. If your arms are not supported, and your back and shoulders remain hunched, over time, you will likely experience pain and tightness in your neck and back.

The "football hold" is also a great position for early breastfeeding, or when breastfeeding twins. In this hold, the baby is tucked under your arm, close to your side, so it is easy to drop your nipple into your baby's wide-open mouth and pull your baby's head toward the breast simultaneously. This position can also require a lot of pillow support for the mother.

A side-lying nursing position may not work well until you and your baby have gotten familiar with upright positions, and until your baby has greater control over his head. Mothers often need to sit up in bed to breastfeed newborns for the first few weeks. Two to six weeks is the average time when side-lying becomes feasible.

Latch

Achieving a good latch is often the hardest part of breastfeeding. Babies born early, and even some full-term babies, have trouble opening their mouths wide enough, sucking hard enough, or coordinating their jaw muscles. With most term babies, this evens out in the first weeks. With premature babies, improvement might not be significant until they are closer to their gestational due date.

A good latch is easy to identify once you've seen one. There are two factors that are critical. The first is whether you are comfortable. If you are in pain, more than a little discomfort, something is not quite right, no matter how many times a nurse or friend says the latch looks great. The second factor is whether the baby is getting milk. We will talk about that in a minute. Usually, the baby's mouth is wide

CORRECT INFANT LATCH-ON

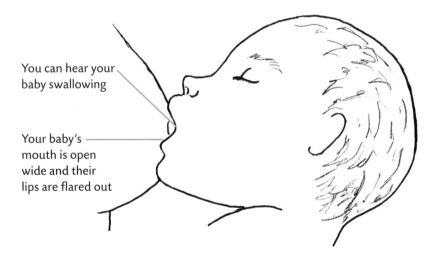

You can hear your baby swallowing

Your baby's mouth is open wide and their lips are flared out

open and both lips are flared out. You can see a small glimpse of pink-ish color inside the baby's mouth, near the edge of the lips, because the lips are spread so far. The bottom lip is not tucked under or curled (a common problem). If this occurs, you can break the latch gently using your pinky finger. Insert your finger at the corner of your baby's mouth to break the suction and then try again.

Another clue that you have attained a good latch is you can hear and see that your baby is swallowing. Your baby can suck without swallowing, so learning the signs of swallowing is helpful, especially at the beginning. When your baby swallows, his jaw will drop downward in a slower, deeper movement than when he is only sucking. You can usually hear a small gulping sound the baby makes when milk is swallowed.

If you hear clicking sounds, these may be an indication that the baby's tongue is curling or retracting, and that the latch is not optimal, especially if you are in pain.

Judging Whether Your Baby is Getting Enough Milk

In the early days you should not be super concerned with whether your baby is drinking enough colostrum. Work on achieving good latches, and put your baby to the breast often. There will not be as much colostrum as there will be milk. Be assured, babies are designed to lose weight for the first 3 to 4 days while you nourish them with the power-house of immunity colostrum provides.

Once your milk comes in, you and your care providers will pay attention to how your baby gains weight. Ideally, your baby will start gaining by the end of the first week, and return to birth weight by ten to fourteen days. However, if you received fluids through an IV during labor or delivery, your baby's "birth weight" is more accurately measured when your baby is twenty-four hours old, according to researchers from the University of Ottawa.

We now know that the IV fluids are absorbed not only by the mother, but the baby, too. So babies can be born weighing several ounces more than truly represents their actual body weight. Just like the mothers, babies need at least a day to shed that extra fluid.

A general rule of thumb is that babies will breastfeed about eight to ten times a day, at a minimum. Some babies will feed more often than that. Most care providers recommend you wake your baby for feedings every two to three hours in the first week or two. It is not the end of the world, *if everything else is looking good* and the rest of the time you adhere to two- to three-hour feedings, to allow a four-hour stretch of sleep at night in the first week.

It's not critical for you to know how much milk you're making, or how much your baby is drinking, once your baby starts to gain weight at a continuous rate. When this happens, you may begin to let your baby sleep for longer stretches of time. If your baby is active and engaged during feeding sessions (not sleepy, lethargic, or too fussy to eat), you will probably find that your baby continues to gain weight even with sleeping sessions lasting many hours. If your baby is sleeping four or five hours at a stretch, you can weigh him every three or four days for the first few weeks to make sure the weight gain is maintained. If it is, be assured your baby is getting enough to eat.

If your baby is not gaining weight at all, or is gaining weight slowly, remember to take in the full picture. After the initial two to four weeks, we expect babies to grow on average an ounce (28 g) a day until weight gain slows around four months. Remember this is an average. Some babies gain more and some gain a bit less. When babies do not follow this path exactly, we must also look at other clues to decide whether this baby is healthy or requires intervention. How many wet and dirty diapers does the baby have in one day? How is the baby's overall look, especially the skin? Are there any signs of dehydration, such as dry mouth, an absence of tears, or sunken eyes? How is the baby's activity level? Is the mother or the father considered petite?

The pediatrician's growth chart is based on *averages* and, if you remember your elementary school math, averages are constructed from a range of data points, some of which are higher or lower than the decided average. Your baby may be well within the range of normal, but possibly closer to either the higher or lower data points. Use all data available—not just the raw numbers—to decide whether your baby's weight gain is enough.

Squirting Milk and Leaking

An unfortunate reality of lactation is the possibility of leaking milk. Stock up on your favorite kind of nursing pad! Just like diapers, nursing pad options have exploded in the last decade. There are colorful, reusable cloth nursing pads on many websites, such as Etsy and Amazon. Yet even the best nursing pad can soak through on one side when you latch your baby onto the other. When I was at home, I often used the standard white diapers on the leaking side to solve this dilemma. Squirting and leaking resolve themselves in a few weeks as your body begins to regulate milk production, creating "on demand" instead of proactively. This regulation takes longest for a first baby and kicks in faster for subsequent babies.

When Breastfeeding Is Challenging

You Are in Pain Contrary to what most of us have been told, it is a myth that breastfeeding should not hurt. I believe it would be more helpful to acknowledge that mild discomfort is common in the first weeks. However, if it gets worse instead of better, reach out for help. Any visible damage to your nipples, such as cracks, cuts, or bleeding, also means you should ask for help. Also, if pain is increasing, not getting better with time, something is not right. Often, a latch correction is possible with a bit of coaching. Remember, breastfeeding will not be sustainable if you are in significant pain, or if your nipples are continually being damaged.

Your Baby Won't Latch On This can be extremely frustrating—for you and your baby. I will venture to say there is likely nothing worse than holding a crying, obviously hungry baby in your arms, and not being able to help her latch and suck properly. This is most likely out of your scope of experience. In this case, seek help from experienced breastfeeding troubleshooters.

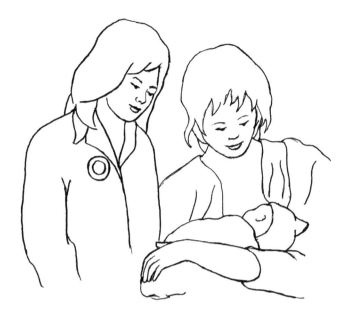

Accessing Breastfeeding Help

In Canada, lactation consultants are often free, and many cities have drop-in clinics. You can find additional support at La Leche League as well. In the United States, you may receive enough support from free groups, such as La Leche League or another community resource; however, you may need to hire an IBCLC. If you are a low-income mother, you may be able to access a free lactation consultant (and a breast pump) through the Women, Infant, and Children (WIC) program.

International board-certified lactation consultants (IBCLCs) have, what I call, "the equivalent of a Ph.D. in lactation." They have studied lactation in depth and know much more about it than physicians (unless a physician has specialized in this area). Even pediatricians do not receive extensive training in breastfeeding and, unless they have gone out of their way to access additional training, do not know the tips and tricks that lactation consultants do. Pediatricians, by nature of their job, are usually more concerned with making sure your baby is getting enough nutrition than they are with troubleshooting breastfeeding challenges (although there are exceptions). IBCLCs are trained to support the mother–baby dyad in difficult lactation circumstances.

When you meet with an IBCLC, you should leave the session feeling more hopeful, not more defeated. This is an accurate measurement of whether this particular IBCLC is a good fit for you. You may decide together that supplementing with donor milk, or formula, is the best option for the moment, but, whatever you decide, you should feel hopeful about the overall plan. Did you identify a goal you believe is worthwhile? Did you work together to brainstorm tangible and realistic steps toward that goal? It's important to find a lactation consultant who believes deeply in breastfeeding and is not willing to give up on the first session.

Be Willing to Go Out of the Western Medicine Comfort Zone to Find Answers
An interesting problem in the developed world is how little support Western medicine offers for breastfeeding challenges. We have loads of scientific studies about how beneficial breastfeeding is for babies and for mothers, yet a dearth of information to help mothers troubleshoot breastfeeding challenges. As I've noted, physicians receive very little training about lactation (about one hour, on average, of lecture in medical school).

One area in which Western medicine is becoming more proactive is evaluating tongue ties in infants. A tongue tie (when the tongue cannot extend far enough out of the mouth for effective sucking action) can be helped by a relatively simple cut. There are few nerve endings in this area, and babies do not often react with strong crying to the procedure. In the past, mothers had to wait through weeks or months of painful breastfeeding until the baby's tongue and mouth grew larger. Yet, today, physicians identify and treat more cases of tongue-tied infants.

Non-Western practices offer many more options for lactation support. In many areas of Western medicine, problems are treated with pharmaceutical drugs. As there are no drugs to help in these situations, and the only helpful solution Western medicine has been able/willing to offer is the tongue-tie procedure, lactation support is an area where even mainstream women explore nonstandard modalities. Remember, it doesn't have to work for everyone to work for you. It is worth trying a variety of ideas, and if something helps, keep doing it—and if it doesn't help, keep looking.

Many mothers praise craniosacral therapy and chiropractic care if a baby is struggling to latch, a mother is in pain, or a baby is not able to transfer enough breastmilk. The idea is that something is not functioning quite right in the baby's musculoskeletal system and is interfering with proper breastfeeding technique. Some find almost immediate relief after an initial session, while others see incremental improvement over time.

Other families have tried acupuncture, Reiki, and infant massage. Mothers can also try different herbs to promote milk supply.

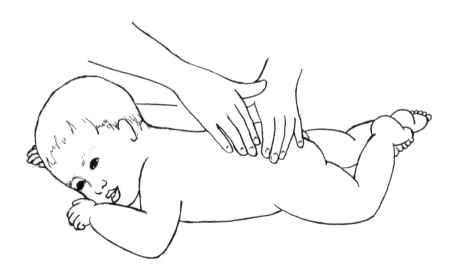

Find a Support Group Mothers experiencing breastfeeding challenges need a support group even more than other mothers. Experiencing pain and frustration around this fundamental part of motherhood can be isolating and depressing. Many communities have free or low-cost breastfeeding support groups. Check out La Leche League International's website for groups near you.

It's Never Too Late to Get Breastfeeding Help

When I struggled with latching pain with my second baby at nine months of age, I stopped by a drop-in breastfeeding clinic in Toronto for help. Even though I had breastfed my oldest and had been breastfeeding my second without problems for nine months, I was still able to benefit from the latching tips I received during this session. Barbara Robertson tells story after story of mothers who learn that beginning to breastfeed at six weeks can be successful, or that it is possible to transition a baby from a bottle back to the breast at eight weeks of age. Don't give up because you think some magic window of time has closed.

If you plan to go back to paid employment in the first twelve weeks after birth, seek out accurate information about breastfeeding, pumping, and working with a nursing infant at home. I offer three tips here to get you started. It's also a good idea to check out the online resources recommended in this chapter.

1. Whoever feeds your baby should learn as much as possible about "paced feeding" (see page 101 for more information). Paced bottle feeding means your baby does not rush through a bottle and finish faster than her body is able to create satiety signals. A feeding should take at least fifteen to twenty minutes, not just a few. Babies who are not being paced bottle-fed run the risk of being under or overfed, experiencing stress during feedings, or even refusing to take the breast.

2. Be aware of how often you remove milk from your breasts. It is not always easy to pump at work, so you may be tempted to skip pumping sessions. There are phone apps to help you keep track of how

many feedings/pumpings happen in a twenty-four-hour period. Generally speaking, you need a minimum of eight milk removals per day to maintain your milk supply. You will become more familiar with your body and your baby as you work through this process.

3. Find a good quality pump if you will depend on pumping to feed your baby while you're working. This may not be the most expensive. Sometimes your insurance company will give you a pump. If it's one that works well for you, that's great. If it does not, consider investing in a better one.

Your Breastfeeding Experience Does Not Have to "Make Up" for Your Birthing Experience

Many women have beautiful, joyful birthing experiences. In all kinds of births, women can feel empowered. They move forward from the event feeling stronger and more capable. A positive birth experience sets a woman up for successful breastfeeding, due in part to the uninterrupted flow of oxytocin. A mother with a positive birthing experience feels good about her baby and the birth, and her feel-good hormones support successful lactation. In addition, she brings to breastfeeding a confidence from her recent empowering physical experience— "If I can handle *that*, I can surely handle *this.*"

Unfortunately, many other women are not able to enjoy the oxytocin and confidence that flow from an empowering birthing experience. Women in the Western world undergo millions of medical interventions during labor every year, including, but not limited to, surgery, epidural injection, induction, augmentation, episiotomy, and the use of forceps or vacuum. Some of these are welcomed, while some are entirely resented. According to the CDC, 32 percent of all births in the United States are by cesarean section. Certainly, a small minority of women proactively choose to have surgical delivery (less than 1 percent), but for most women, a cesarean birth is not their ideal. Other women, even if they achieved an unmedicated vaginal birth, experienced distress because of unexpected events, such as painful tears or hemorrhage.

Cesarean Statistics

It's important to know that at gestational age thirty-nine weeks (forty weeks is the mythical "due date"), 36 percent of mothers delivered by cesarean in 2015 (trending upward from the 2009 number of 34 percent). This is, presumably, because so many doctors induce women between thirty-eight and thirty-nine weeks, and inductions are more likely to lead to cesareans than are spontaneous labors.

It is understandable that 3 to 17 percent of mothers are estimated to suffer from post-traumatic stress related to their baby's birth. Many more women do not meet diagnostic criteria for PTSD (post-traumatic stress disorder), but, nonetheless, feel disappointment or feelings of failure about their labor or delivery.

Women who are disappointed about how their baby's birth progressed do not get to reap the helpful benefits of an empowering birth experience: uninterrupted oxytocin flow and confidence. Instead, their confidence in their body's ability to feed their baby may be deeply shaken. If they trusted their body in birth and it "failed" them, won't it fail again? One way women compensate for this perceived failure is by turning breastfeeding into a quest for a Holy Grail. They may think unconsciously, or say aloud quite deliberately, "I must succeed in breastfeeding my baby to make up for the way the birth went." Unfortunately, this attitude sometimes backfires and produces more pain and more feelings of failure, especially if the new mother is judging breastfeeding as a pass/fail experience.

So, how can you move past the trauma of a difficult birth to embrace the journey of breastfeeding a newborn? Ideas include making conscious time and space for processing your baby's birth story, asking yourself how you would approach the current breastfeeding session or breastfeeding challenge if you had achieved your ideal birth, and celebrating all the progress you make toward your goals, no matter how small. Getting good lactation support is also very helpful. You don't have to do this alone.

At mother–baby groups, many mothers are articulate about this connection between how they feel about breastfeeding and how they feel about their birthing experience. As the baby cries at her breast, frustrated or unable to latch well, the mother cries, too, saying, as Jeannie of Ann Arbor, Michigan, said once, "I just want something to go right!"

Surprisingly, asking this mother how she thinks she would handle this same scenario *had she given birth the way she desired* results in squared shoulders, raised head, and increased confidence. She realizes she would, very likely, approach challenges the same way, and seek the same advice, but with more confidence. As Jeannie answered, "I would just feel better because I would know I could trust my body." So we asked her, "But what if you were facing the exact situation? Your baby is

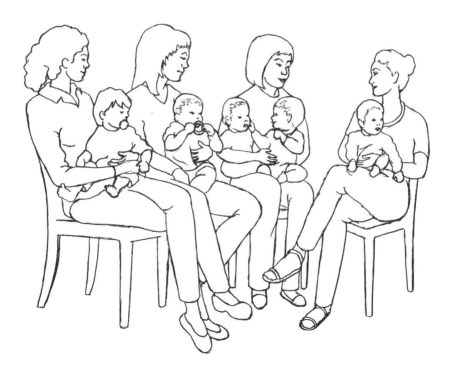

crying and having trouble with his latch." She said, "I would just believe it would work out eventually." Then she got a big smile on her face and said, "Oh. I get it! It's the same situation whether I had a good birth or not. So, I can have confidence or not. I would have to figure it out right now even if I didn't get an epidural." The rest of that day, Jeannie seemed significantly calmer. When she came back the next week, she announced continued improvement in her baby's latch, but also in her outlook regarding their breastfeeding future.

Your birth experience is important—it *is* tied to your breastfeeding experience. However, you still have the ability to release the blame and guilt and "Holy Grail" questing. Beating yourself up only makes you less patient with the process. Be gentle with yourself, and focus on incremental steps toward a better latch, an increased milk supply, or more successful feeding sessions.

Other Means of Infant Feeding

Although breastfeeding may conjure a cozy picture of a mother cradling an infant across her lap, many breastfeeding mothers cannot feed their babies at the breast for every feeding. Other mothers, for a number of reasons, may find that formula-feeding is the right choice for their baby or situation. In these cases, milk or formula is delivered through finger-feeding, cup-feeding, or bottle-feeding. Read on to learn more.

Finger-Feeding and Cup-Feeding

If you intend to breastfeed exclusively, or in combination with bottle-feeding, plan to avoid bottles for the first six weeks if possible. This gives your infant ample time to establish solid breastfeeding habits before being introduced to artificial nipples.

Some babies have no trouble switching back and forth from bottle to breast, but others come to prefer the flow of bottles. We used to call this "nipple confusion," but we now know it is not nipple confusion, but flow preference. This is another reason that paced bottle feeding is

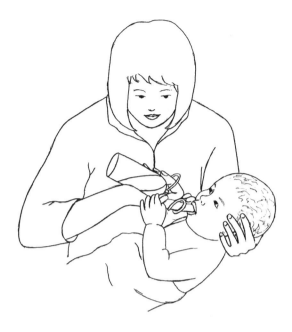

so important. It slows the flow and makes bottle feeding work more like breastfeeding.

If you need to be away from your baby for a feeding during these first weeks before you've introduced a bottle, there are other methods you can use, such as finger- or cup-feeding. Finger-feeding uses a tube taped to an adult's finger. Online retailers sell the equipment (also called a "supplemental nursing/feeding system") and it is not too expensive. Cup-feeding is just what it sounds like: using a small container, such as the medicine cups that come with many over-the-counter liquid medicines. You sit your infant up on your lap, and put the cup to the edge of her bottom lip so she can drink it. The adult does not need to pour the milk into the baby's mouth; the baby is able to lap it up from the cup. If this sounds like a method you want to try, there are helpful videos online that give you a visual image of how it works. I recommend the series of videos available at: Breast-feeding.support/cup-feeding-newborn.

Bottle-Feeding

If you are ready to try bottle-feeding your baby, the most critical piece of information to retain is the importance of pacing your baby's intake. When you imagine bottle-feeding, you may picture a baby being held in a horizontal position and a bottle that is nearly vertical. This position means your baby guzzles milk, without any breaks, and likely drinks more than he would otherwise.

Paced bottle-feeding is a method that allows babies to eat slowly and recognize the feeling of satiety. This mimics the breastfeeding experience more closely.

In paced bottle-feeding, the baby is held more upright on your lap, while the bottle is held horizontally to slow milk flow. The baby is allowed to suck the nipple into his own mouth and begin the feeding, rather than having the nipple tipped into his mouth forcefully. The baby should do most of the work. There is more information about this method on page 101. Videos are available online through the Breast-Feeding Center of Ann Arbor at youtube.com/watch?v=1cvF1nawMNI, and from the Pennsylvania-based Breast-Feeding Resource Center at youtube.com/watch?v=dxpIzcitLc8.

Preparing to Return to Paid Employment as a Breastfeeding Mother

A hot topic at mother–baby groups is always the preparation for returning to paid employment. In Canada, where I gave birth to my second child, parents have one year of paid leave that can be split between two parents in any way (so, for example, the birth mother can take off ten months and her partner can take off two). In the United States, women are lucky if they have twelve weeks of unpaid leave, if they're working for a large employer or a generous small business. The majority of American women (88 percent) are not even allowed these twelve weeks. A stunning 23 percent of American women go back to work *ten days or sooner* after having a baby.

Although I am very aware of the financial pressures correlated with taking time out of the paid workforce (these pressures were strong in my own family), I believe new mothers often need a sense of permission to entertain any thought of extending their parental leave. So, if you are feeling any stress about going back to your job, I encourage you to take a hard look at all your options. If your goal is to breastfeed, it is important to establish a positive, good breastfeeding relationship with your baby before you go back to work, if possible. Premature babies, especially, may be somewhat "behind" their full-term counterparts when the average twelve weeks of leave ends. Starting with a functioning breastfeeding relationship strengthens the possibility of successful pumping and breastfeeding going forward.

What you planned to do before your baby arrives may continue to be a great plan after, but it doesn't hurt to reevaluate your plans either. Ask yourself what is the optimal childcare/paid employment situation for all members of your family. If you faced any birth or baby challenges that made the first weeks stressful, you or your partner might consider taking unpaid leave you hadn't considered before. A few extra weeks of a parent being at home might help relieve some stress. The best answer might be rearranging work schedules for both of you, or inviting a family member, such as a grandparent, to stay for a few months; or even extending your leave. One father reported he took Fridays off work for twelve weeks after his partner went back to work. Many parents find a gradual return to work (a few days a week or half days) is easier than the standard all-or-nothing plan.

Still, at some point, you may find yourself going back to a paid job and entrusting your baby to someone else's care. During the fourth trimester, you will need to hire that caregiver and start pumping breastmilk for your freezer supply, if you intend to maintain breastfeeding. It is also a good idea to find out when and where you can pump while at work.

Studies show the majority of women who need to pump outside their home do not feel they have a safe place to do so. This is one reason so many mothers end up in bathroom stalls—at least the doors have a lock. In an ideal world, there would be a safe, private, and comfortable place for you to pump at work. You would have access to an electrical outlet, and a refrigerator or freezer to store your pumped milk (although, an insulated cooler with ice packs can also safely hold your milk for up to twenty-four hours). In the United States, businesses with more than fifty employees have to provide a space (that is not a bathroom) to pump and time to pump. This is a legal obligation under federal law. For more information, see www.dol.gov/whd/nursingmothers.

How Long Pumped Breastmilk Lasts

AT ROOM TEMERPATURE	IN THE REFRIGERATOR	IN THE FREEZER
4 to 8 hours	Fresh milk: 3 to 8 days Thawed milk: 24 hours	3 to 6 months Store at the back of the freezer for deepest freeze
TIP: It's okay to add fresh breastmilk to frozen breastmilk, just keep the date of the older milk. Freeze milk in small batches, perhaps 1 to 3 fluid ounces (30 to 90 ml), so you only have to thaw what you need.		

The Freezer Stash Mothers, sometimes, are overly concerned with building up a large stash of breastmilk in the freezer, and helping their baby learn to use a bottle *before* they go back to work. However, at twelve weeks postpartum, many mothers are still recovering from giving birth, not getting enough sleep, starting to think about having sex with their partner again, and don't really have time to pump. Establishing stable breastfeeding habits while nurturing a deep connection with baby is most important. Many women return to paid employment without as much milk in the freezer as they had hoped.

Undoubtedly, it is a great idea to begin building a stash four weeks or so before you plan to return to work. You may only get one to two ounces (60 ml) at a time, but eventually it adds up. The ideal time to

Paced Bottle-Feeding, by Barbara Robertson, IBCLC

Pacing the bottle-feed helps:

- Babies feel safe and comfortable while they feed
- Keep the flow more like breastfeeding
- Reduce overfeeding babies with a bottle
- Protect the breastfeeding relationship

How pacing the feed works:

- Have the baby sit upright.
- Use a slow-flow, wide-based bottle teat.
- Touch the baby's chin or upper lip with the tip of the teat. When the baby cues for feeding by opening her mouth, gently slide the teat in as deeply as the baby allows.
- Hold the bottle so the breastmilk just fills the teat.
- Don't worry about the baby swallowing air. You may need to burp more, but this is a small price for baby adapting to easy feeding. We want to teach babies that feeding takes time and effort, with the breast, and with the bottle.
- After about three swallows, gently twist the teat so the nipple seal is broken and rest the teat against the baby's chin, cheek, or upper lip. This allows the baby to catch her breath, to realize feeding takes time, and to learn not to worry that the breastmilk and bottle are gone.
- Is baby getting stressed? Is she frowning, wrinkling her forehead, widening her eyes, splaying her hands, making squeaking sounds, choking? If so, twist the teat out of her mouth and give her a break.
- When she cues again by opening her mouth wide, repeat the process.

This process should take about twenty minutes. Babies need time to realize they are full, just like adults. It takes time, but it is so worth it!

Watch for satiety cues: becoming sleepy, not opening the mouth, turning away from the teat, seeming more interested in surroundings. Let her decide when she is done. If you feel the baby has had an appropriate amount of supplement, take a break, have a burp, change a diaper, shift position, and see if the baby cues again.

pump is after your baby has breastfed. Generally, mothers make more milk in the morning than the evening, so you might try pumping after a morning feed if you are only pumping once a day, or after one morning feed and one evening feed if you are pumping twice a day. Your goal might be to save enough milk for one week of childcare, but if you can get enough milk for even two or three days, you may be able to stay on top of the supply.

The trick is to find the right rhythm at work as soon as possible. This way, you are pumping the same amount of milk your baby is drinking while you are away from each other. It's important for your childcare provider to understand the importance of paced feedings so you don't go through your frozen milk too quickly.

You may discover your baby feeds more in the evenings and through the night after you return to work. Cluster feeding in the evening is common. This is when you sit on your couch for two hours or more while your baby feeds off and on for what feels like forever. It's helpful if your partner is supportive and aware this might happen. Your partner may end up doing a lot more cooking, cleaning, and laundry, but will also be helping preserve the breastfeeding relationship. Many mothers also find their babies create their own schedules to optimize their time at the breast.

Conclusion

Taking care of a newborn, especially your first, is an enormous adjustment. As one new father remarked to me, "If someone told you that you'd have to squeeze a second twenty-hour-a-week job into your already full life, you'd tell them it's impossible. There's literally no space for that. But babies require even more time. It's impossible, but somehow we all do it." Maybe you have taken care of a pet, or added a big responsibility to your life before, but it is rarely the kind of responsibility that can demand attention from you at any moment in a twenty-four-hour period for years at a time.

The nature of parenthood makes most of us willing to sacrifice our own well-being for the sake of our children; however, knowing how to do this in a sustainable way is important. I find it helpful to remember that taking care of myself is good parenting, even if my child is disappointed in the moment. You are modeling positive self-care so children will later know how to take care of themselves.

You will master all the other topics I mentioned relatively quickly: bathing, diapering, and even infant feeding. Even though you may struggle with breastfeeding challenges or feeling confident your baby is growing well over time, I predict that self-care will remain the largest challenge you face as a parent. Remember that your baby—and, later, older child—has an insatiable appetite for your time and attention. Remember, also, that children are resilient, and will learn to do what they see you doing—whether it be running around like crazy with no time for yourself, or intentionally making time for the things you enjoy.

You are doing a hard job for which you will get very little credit. However, do not doubt that what you are doing is valuable. What you impart to your children will, literally, become the future of humanity. That alone is worth a deep breath, a step back, and a conscious decision to support the other parents around you in their hard work, too.

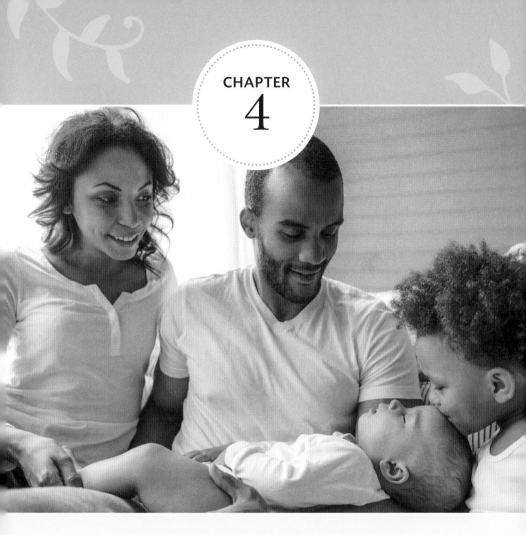

CHAPTER
4

YOUR CHANGING RELATIONSHIPS WITH YOUR IMMEDIATE FAMILY: PARTNER, CHILDREN, AND PETS

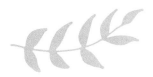

N O HUMAN BABY IS BORN INTO A SOCIAL VACUUM. Every baby is born into a web of relationships. Relationships can be challenging to manage when there are only two partners —they are even trickier with more people involved. Sometimes, our instincts help us navigate relationships well. Other times, we greatly benefit from putting conscious thought and effort into nurturing a particular relationship. As you bring a baby into your home, you will probably notice ripple effects among the immediate family. This chapter explores ways we relate differently with partners, older children, and even our pets, while we simultaneously parent a newborn.

If you do not have a partner, an older child, or a dog, feel free to skip ahead. If you are co-parenting but not living together, you might still enjoy the short section about letting your partner make his or her own way as a parent.

Your Changing Relationship with Your Partner

Family is all about love. In these early months, however, staying connected to your partner may become much harder than you ever imagined. If this is your first baby, you've never had to share responsibilities together quite

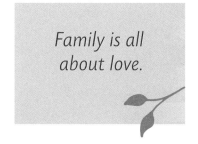

Family is all about love.

like this, and you've probably never had to navigate your romantic relationship around another human being's demanding schedule. If this is not your first child, you are used to the juggling—oh, but now you are experiencing so much more of it! You may have previously enjoyed an active sex life before having a baby, and even used sex as a means of reconciling day-to-day stresses. This becomes much harder with a baby. Sex itself is such a significant issue that I've allotted it space in chapter 6 (see page 163). Here, you can explore other ways to stay close to your partner.

Maintaining intimacy and connection with your partner while you navigate the fourth trimester of having a new baby is not easy, but it is well worth any effort you give. In fact, having a baby together may be one of the most common pathways toward a more mature relationship. By mature relationship, I mean sharing a deep connection firmly rooted in knowing one another well—flaws and all. Couples who do not have children are not always forced toward this level of maturity, so it can take them longer to attain it.

So, here's some bad news. According to the *Denver Post* (April 9, 2009), "Having a kid puts a sudden, drastic strain on a marriage" or partnership. They write that *90 percent* of couples report significant dips in marital satisfaction during the first year of parenthood. The Relationship Research Institute finds that 13 percent of parents married at the time of having a baby, get divorced within five years; 39 percent of unmarried couples who have a baby split within the same period. Perhaps least surprising, parents report less satisfaction with their financial situation compared to nonparents. This is all sobering news.

I think it is helpful to know that many complications of the first year of parenthood are unavoidable. How you respond to them matters most, but it is unlikely you will be able to sidestep the new challenges in your relationship that need addressing. For example, who, exactly, will be the one to have an uninterrupted eight hours of sleep every night? This is a common question many couples face early on. Who will be in charge of taking your children to the doctor? Who will handle the extra loads of laundry? This chapter offers tips for maintaining a solid connection with your significant other; however, you cannot hope to avoid these relationship trials. The challenges of new parenthood are not anyone's fault and, unfortunately, they are not optional.

At the start of your relationship, especially when you began living together, you had to solve many different problems, yet you faced these troubles in the glow of new love, or even infatuation. Parenthood has a way of stripping away any rose-colored glasses that previously allowed us to see each other in only the most positive light. Now, you must solve mutual issues while you are sleep-deprived, while a baby is crying, or while you are trying to keep the baby asleep. These are not ideal conditions for two adults to engage in rational conversation and problem solving.

Be encouraged: I have good news, too. Although many people cite having a child as the reason for divorce, the truth is that couples with children are about 40 percent *less likely* to divorce than couples without children. Although parents appear to be less satisfied with their financial situation than nonparents, parents are more satisfied with their overall family life.

Tips for Staying Close to Your Partner

1. Remember, even when each of you gives 100 percent as parents, there will still be a gap to fill.

2. Accept help and hire help.

3. Go out by yourself (especially you, new mother!).

4. Let each person parent their own way, even if it makes you or your partner crazy.

5. Remember, "Date Night" doesn't have to mean going out.

6. Say "Thank you" to each other every day.

If you can maintain a loving and open attitude toward your partner, there is every chance that, on the other side of this challenging time, you will discover you are more in love than ever. You will have created meaningful family rituals. You will have learned that in the loneliness of selflessly taking care of a baby, you can count on each other. You will have survived seeing each other in unflattering situations. You will know your partner still finds you attractive despite the stretch marks and scars. There is great emotional intimacy that comes from sharing vulnerability and pain. Out of this shared experience, you can create a deeper bond than you had before. Here are some tips to help you arrive at this destination.

Remember, Even When Each of You Gives 100 Percent as Parents, There Will Still Be a Gap to Fill

I learned this pointer from parent-educator Catherine Fisher, one of the doulas in my doula partnership, Tree Town Doulas. When she says this, she draws in the air with two hands. One hand represents the new mother's 100 percent effort. The other hand represents her partner's 100 percent effort. Between them, she leaves a large gap. Even though I knew this intellectually, seeing the truth in this visual format helped me internalize it.

Take a moment to dwell on this thought for a few moments because this one insight alone can change everything. Instead of being mad at your partner because something important has been left undone, you can share your unhappiness at the impossibility of getting everything done well when you have small children. Instead of blaming the love of your life, you can hold each other in appreciation for what does get done.

In the past, in Western culture and in many places today, extended family fills in this gap. If you live near helpful family members you know what I mean. When a parent stays up with a sick child at night, a sibling might stop by with a meal or an uncle might mow your lawn. A friend, who lived near both sets of grandparents, was blessed with overnight childcare once a week for many years, starting as soon as she was willing to separate from her babies overnight. It was great for her children to get to know their grandparents well, and it was amazing for my friend, who was able to take care of herself and her relationship in a relaxed way.

Two adults are simply not capable of doing all that needs to be done when you add children to the picture. Keeping this truth in the forefront of your mind will help you be more patient with each other. You can talk about how to handle those things that fall into the gap between your 100-percents with less blame and anger. There is a huge difference between hearing your loved one say, "Why didn't you fill the dishwasher before you left for work?" and "I've noticed one thing we can't do consistently every day is the dishes. I know you are giving your all right now and you're really tired, too. I feel the same way. I don't know how we're going to fix this problem. Will you help me think of ways we can make sure this is a priority so it doesn't stack up on us?" Aim for the latter and your relationship will grow instead of suffer.

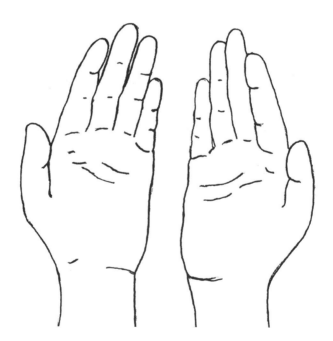

Keeping in mind that there will always be a gap to fill even when both parents give 100 percent can help parents be more patient with one another.

Accept Help and Hire Help

Things that fall into this natural gap are housework and cooking. If you can, find a third party to help. Relatives and friends often are a first place to turn. This is no time to be a superhero. Accept any assistance that makes your life easier. Solicit help. Hire help. As Ayesha, a mother of three, reports, "I never paid someone to clean my house before. It's my house. Why would I let someone else clean it? But after the twins arrived, my husband and I were fighting about housecleaning all the time. Finally, I just decided it was cheaper to pay for a cleaning service than to pay for a divorce." Hiring help is, indeed, expensive, yet peace of mind can sometimes be worth it.

Go Out by Yourself (Especially You, New Mother!)

Ruddy has a fabulous list of suggestions at Parenting.com for making your love relationship work after having children. She agrees with me that making time for yourself, away from your baby, is a surprise key ingredient to keeping a strong connection to your partner. She writes, "You can't be each other's only outlet, so find other ones. Having a life outside your family will make you a better wife and a better mother and a better person." This, by the way, helps you have something to talk about with your significant other *besides* how often your baby pooped that day.

Let Each Person Parent Their Own Way, Even if It Makes You or Your Partner Crazy

In 2000 when I worked at a Russian birth hospital, the mothers gave birth without their partners and stayed at the hospital for five days (after a vaginal birth), or two weeks (after a cesarean). Partners spray-painted messages to the mothers on a wall outside the hospital and sent baskets of goodies, but they often did not meet their new babies face to face until the mothers left the hospital. I became aware that those days of isolation were enough to make birth mothers "experts" in baby care compared to their partners, and I could never shake the feeling these families were set up for an unequal sharing of childcare responsibilities. When I interviewed Russians about gender and childcare, I was often told, "mothers are naturally more capable" in this area.

I don't believe there is a gender gene for childcare, but I do see how this capability grows more quickly within the parent who does the majority of the childcare work. Only a small fraction of Western families enjoy perfect parity in work–family time; usually one parent spends more time with a baby than another. That parent, naturally, becomes more attuned to the baby's needs and preferences. You could say this parent ends up doing things "better" than the other one.

However, if you are the parent with more experience at the beginning, just because you might be able to do things more efficiently than your partner doesn't mean you shouldn't allow your partner to bungle through on her own. It's okay to occasionally share helpful suggestions ("I've found she cries less if you burp her every five minutes," for example), but too much advice can push you into controlling territory—and harm your partner's confidence in parenting. Instead of explaining how to take care of your child, take a deep breath and get out of the way. Toni Auker, another of my doula partners, offers this story:

> I worked as a server until my second child was born. I chose to work closing shifts so my son would be home with Daddy instead of a sitter. I realized, pretty early on, I couldn't dictate how he did bedtime. As my go-to solution was nursing him to sleep, he would need to find his own way. He might have let him stay up later, watch more TV, or eat a late-night snack, but when I got home they were both sound asleep. Almost six years later, I never worry about going out at night. I know they will have fun and will probably go to bed better than normal nights.

Louise, another mother from Michigan, describes how her husband's approach to dressing their daughter was a blessing in disguise she was able to appreciate years later.

*When we ran a family business, my daily shift at the store was
6 a.m. to 4 p.m., so I, literally, never dressed my daughter for school
or anything from two years on. My ex-husband, bless his heart, was
only interested in making sure she was wearing one top, one bottom,
two socks, and two shoes. He let our daughter choose them herself.*

*Up until that time, I had dressed her in items that at least looked
like they belonged together—and facing the right direction. What
ensued was great joy in dressing, which became free expression
unhindered by societal expectation. She is nineteen now and still
employs this free expression daily.*

*If I were there, I might have dampened her enthusiasm—with
things like rules. The few times I had a chance to dress her in those
young years, I put her in some outfit that "matched," and, honestly,
it never looked right on her. She usually changed by lunchtime. Her
style was established by age four. I think it was mostly her, but it was
also her dad, who let her become herself.*

The short-term benefit of telling your partner what to do is that something will get done your way. It might even, objectively, be the better way, but that's beside the point I want to make. The long-term benefit of letting other adults figure out parenting on their own is that *they figure out parenting on their own.* The faster you learn how to be okay with this, the happier you both will be.

"Date Night" Doesn't Have to Mean Going Out

A regular date night is a great idea to help couples stay connected. After you set aside time for yourself, consciously set aside time for the two of you, too. The truth is, babysitters cancel, and infants can be hard to leave for multiple hours. So, get creative—what can you do to have a weekly date night at home? Changing the vibe from ordinary to special can be as simple as adding candles to dinnertime or setting a rule: "No talk about the baby for the next hour."

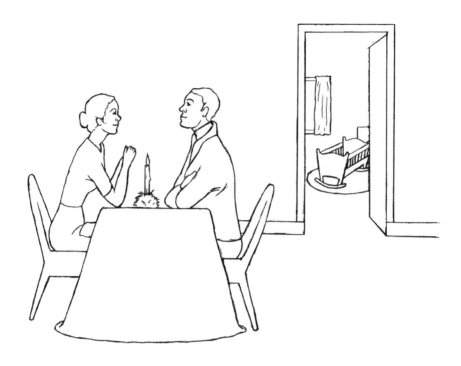

Say "Thank You" to Each Other Every Day

Relationship expert John Gottman found that couples who stay together have five times as many positive interactions as they do negative interactions. It was likely easy for you and your partner to reach this 5:1 benchmark while dating. It is much harder to do when parenting. However, you can deliberately find a time and place to tell your partner something that you appreciate. Do what you can to increase the number of positive interactions. The authors Les and Leslie Parrott write that consciously cultivating gratitude toward each other works because, "When two people are committed to seeing and appreciating life's gifts together, their perspectives change and broaden. Anxiety tends to lessen, and shared enjoyment increases."

Your Changing Relationship with Your Older Child

What a gift you are giving your older children! Siblings are life-long companions who intuitively understand where each other is coming from because they came from the same place. Although you may have some tap dancing to do in the years ahead to help them live more-or-less peaceably in the same house, you can have hope for their adult years. That is when they truly reap the benefits of a sibling.

There are pros and cons, of course, to having more than one child, and choosing to have only one child may be a smart choice for many parents. In the case of first or only children, you have no sibling relationships to manage, so in this chapter, I focus on the advantages of having siblings. There is no need to discuss the drawbacks if you've already made the decision to have more than one.

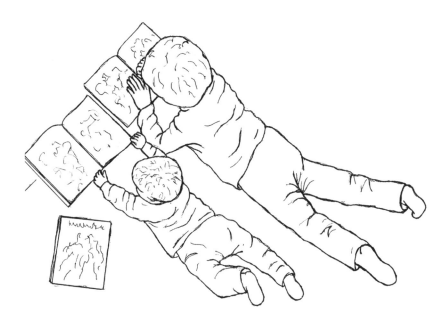

Many of us today did not come from large families, and may have been an only child. New mothers might feel anxious about giving each child enough time and attention and can feel guilty about taking something away from a first child. Despite these normal misgivings, you can find confidence that your choice to have more children is good for you, and good for your children, too.

The Positive Side of Life with Brothers and Sisters

I am an advocate of flipping "sibling guilt" entirely on its head. The potential bonds of friendship, support, and shared responsibility toward the older generation more than tip the balance against the loss of attention received from parents during childhood. It doesn't always turn out perfectly, and certainly there are families in which siblings do not get along, even in adulthood; however, the potential companionship and understanding that siblings can offer to each other is an amazing gift.

If you are an adult who came from a large family, like I did, you may have had a different experience. Some older children do end up resenting their siblings because they had to take on childcare and household responsibilities. Maybe they feel neglected by parents who can't tend to everyone, or perhaps they do not grow up with close family bonds. Even so, my general experience when meeting other members of large families is that we share a positive experience that people from smaller families cannot understand.

Wherever I go, I ask people from large families how they think their childhood has influenced their own parenting. One of the most common responses I receive is they were less afraid than their peers to have children because they already knew and understood what life with babies was all about.

Janine, from Sweetwater, Oklahoma, wrote about this in the Facebook group, Natural Parenting 101:

I grew up in a large family! My dad has three biological kids and two stepkids and my mom had four biological kids and two stepkids. We also had foster kids in and out constantly. My mom breastfed and was very open about everything. None of us was shy growing up. I definitely feel like the fact that there were so many of us made it so much easier to have kids and not feel as much mom guilt. I was the oldest, so when my brother was born, it was my entire world. I never felt left out. I saw my mom mess up and saw how she handled us differently and I think that's what made me the confident mommy I am today!

If you are like most Western women nowadays, you do not plan to have five or seven or ten children. You plan to have one or two or three. I know a handful of families in my circle with four children and have one close friend who is the mother of eight. This variation boils down to a national average of 1.14 children per woman. There are certainly good reasons for this noticeable shift in average family size, including the population size across the globe; however, I think we lose something important as a culture when the majority of children grow up without many siblings.

Giving your child a sibling gives them the rare gift of effortless familiarity with day-to-day life involving babies, toddlers, and small children. Siblings gain an understanding of how to share resources with other people. Giving and receiving in families with more than one child is not just vertical, from the older generation to the younger, but also horizontal, within the children's generation.

When I was a teenager, changing a poopy diaper was as natural as singing the latest hit song. I grew up a witness to successful breastfeeding. I enjoyed holidays from the perspective of a child (all these presents for me!), and from the perspective of a helper to the adults creating magical experiences for my still-young siblings. I loved planning scavenger hunts and decorating cakes for their birthdays. Equally important, I learned I could be extremely different from another person, and go through periods of intense dislike yet still hold a strong bond. The sister closest in age to me has a very different personality from mine, which did not work out so well when we were in middle and high school. However, as adults, we became close. Even though she lives across the world, I "talk" (text, email, or message) with her almost every day.

Of course, siblings in childhood and adulthood go through times when they are closer and times when they are less so. This is less noticeable in large families because, when you are not getting along with one, you can turn to another. When my sister and I were having children at the same time, I reached out to her more than I did our other siblings. Friends who only have one or two siblings experience periods of closeness or more distance, as well, but without any "fill-in-the-gap" siblings. For example, one close friend was not close with her brother at all until their mother died. Now, in their mutual concern about their father, they talk to each more than ever.

Learning how to share toys and attention, to fight and make up with a peer, and how to negotiate, are skills that siblings teach one another better than schools. Having a sibling can be a wonderful thing. If this was not your experience, you may want to reach out to friends for support to help you understand and believe this—in the interest of your own children's happiness and harmony.

I am elaborating on the benefits of having siblings because your own beliefs will undeniably come through in your behavior. If you are solid in your belief that this new baby is a *good thing* for your older child(ren), you will communicate this through your voice, words, and body language. Your older child(ren) will believe you because you are the trustworthy adult. They have no reason to think that a new baby will be a burden or a difficult experience. They know what you tell them and what your actions tell them.

If you are nervous or feel guilty about the additional person coming into your family, your older children will pick up on this subconsciously. They might sense there is something "not quite right" about having a younger sibling. This is likely not the message you intend to broadcast.

I urge you to speak with great confidence about this amazing thing—a brother or sister—coming into their life. You can be truthful about how the new baby won't be able to play right away, and how normal life may become more difficult or different, but you can also speak about the many things they will be able to do together someday.

Tips for Making a Positive Transition for Older Siblings

Here are some tips to help you navigate the beginning weeks and months of having more than one child.

- Focus explanations on the older child.
- Welcome regressive behavior.
- Name the older child's feelings without blaming the baby.
- Create rituals that include your older child.
- Expect the older sibling to wake the baby—a lot!
- Plan ahead for situations in which the baby gets hurt.
- Get support for yourself.
- Enjoy your family.

Focus Explanations on the Older Child Your older child is always more interested in hearing stories about him than about the new baby. When he asks, "Why is the baby upset in the car?" tell a story about your older child as a baby, when *he* cried in the car (made yellow poo in diapers, peed on Daddy's arm, spit up all the time, could only fall asleep in a swing, etc.).

Often, this focus works like magic. Even when it doesn't, keep using it. The older child will learn empathy for the baby by seeing himself in the baby's situation. Otherwise, if you explain from the new baby's perspective, the older child remains focused on his current reaction, which is not necessarily empathetic.

Welcome Regressive Behavior! Regressive behavior, meaning the older child looks like she is going backward in maturity, is not only natural, it is necessary. As I explained, older children develop empathy for their baby sibling by seeing themselves in the baby's situation. This means they might re-explore what it feels like to wet their pants, cry for Mommy/Daddy at nighttime, try breastfeeding again, use a bottle instead of a cup, suck their finger or a pacifier, etc. Children are "playing" what they see the baby doing. They are smart. They see that these behaviors get their parents' attention, so it's worth a try, isn't it? Or perhaps they are sweetly recalling not long ago when these behaviors were satisfying to them and testing to confirm that they are not that interesting anymore.

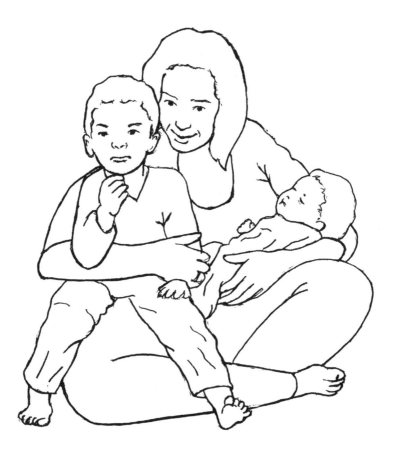

Because we parents have, usually, moved on happily from these dependent stages (welcoming the day when our children learn to use the toilet or give up sucking their thumb), it makes sense we are chagrined to see these behaviors again. However, we will have more success at moving beyond them again if we *welcome* the regressive behavior and overindulge it, rather than punish it or shame our children. (Shaming would be saying something like, "You're a big girl. Big girls don't wet their pants.")

Instead, feel the lump of anger or disappointment rise in your throat, swallow hard, and try this (in as genuine a manner as you can muster): "Oh! How cute! I remember when you were so little and you had to use a diaper all the time! Do you remember when you were too little to use the potty? Let's clean up this pee. Then, do you want to do more things like when you were a baby? What else do you remember from when you were little?" If you interpret each regressive behavior as a sign that your child is trying to develop empathy for the baby, then it is easy to indulge him and help him move through it by "playing baby."

Finally, by welcoming "baby play" so warmly, without shame, your child learns that it's okay to ask for time to be "the baby," rather than doing something like wet his pants to get that kind of parental attention.

One mother relates:

> My daughter LOVES to play "being born." There is a play script we've developed over time. She hides under my shirt and I am supposed to say, "Oh! I feel this baby moving! I wonder if it is a boy or a girl. I wonder when it is going to come out. It's nighttime. I'm going to sleep!" Because she was born at 2:05 a.m., she assumes I was asleep when she arrived! Then she wriggles out, I hold her and coo over her. I give her a name and tell her, "Oh, I've been waiting so long for you to come! I'm so happy to see you!" Whenever she initiates this game, I assume she needs attention and I try to indulge her right away, or as soon as I can.

When your older children feel welcome to the same kind of attention the baby receives, they do not have to resent or feel jealous of their new sibling.

Name the Older Child's Feelings without Blaming the Baby

This is a tough one, but well worth the mental effort! Many sibling preparation books tell us to help older children name their feelings. This is wonderful; however, I suggest we avoid connecting any negative feelings with the baby. The problem is not the baby, per se, but that the older child wants *your* attention. So keep the focus on what your older child wants and needs, and not on the baby's role in the situation. Those feelings and needs are valid. See the box on the opposite page for examples of how to talk about conflicts without blaming the newborn.

Create Rituals that Include Your Older Child

Rituals can make ordinary events feel special. Lighting candles at dinnertime and lowering the lights make dinner feel magical. Invite this magic into your home every day by being creative. This will not only help the older child, it will help you, too. If you create a ritual around changing a diaper, giving the baby a bath, giving the baby a massage, reading the baby a book, etc., you turn these moments into something you look forward to, rather than a chore. What if you change every diaper during the day by candlelight? What if you always open a bottle of lavender oil and give your older child a dab with a cotton ball before you feed the baby? What if bedtime with the older child always includes the question, "What do you remember about (baby's name) today?"

You can assign a delightful responsibility to your older children so they look forward to helping with baby care. I know one mother who found it frustrating to get two small children into car seats multiple times a day. Her ingenious solution was to keep a small spray bottle of flower essences, designed for calming strong feelings, inside her car. Whenever she was putting on the baby's seatbelt, her older daughter got to spritz herself and the baby. She loved spraying the scent, and getting into the car became a happy time instead of a struggle.

Expect the Older Sibling to Wake the Baby—a Lot!

Though it is a good idea to teach your older child skills to help the baby sleep—to use a quiet voice, quiet feet, and quiet toys—teaching this skill is very different than *expecting* your older child to have this skill. Your older

Talking about Conflict

SCENARIO ONE:

Older sibling is whiny and upset because Mommy is breastfeeding the baby AGAIN and she wants to do a puzzle.

Instead of saying, "I see you are mad because I'm with the baby again. I know it seems like all I do is feed the baby. But I will be able to do the puzzle in just a few minutes."

Try: "I see you are feeling mad. You want to do the puzzle right now and I can't. It's really hard to wait and you don't want to wait. I agree it doesn't feel good to have to wait. I'll be able to do the puzzle in just a few minutes."

This way, you do not link the feeling of being mad to anything about the baby, but to *your* inability to play right now.

SCENARIO TWO:

The older child wants you to give her a piggyback ride up the stairs while you are carrying the baby.

Instead of saying, "I can't carry both of you at the same time! You're the big kid so you have to walk."

Try: "Oh, I love giving you piggy back rides! Let me put the baby upstairs on the bed and then I can give you a ride. Oh, I'm so excited!"

Or (if you just have to say no): "Oh, I love giving you piggy back rides! Remember when I carried you all over the zoo that way? I wonder if there is a hippopotamus under my shoe. Will you check under my shoes when I take each step?"

Again, whatever you say, you are not linking the older child's feelings of disappointment to the baby.

child *does not already have* this skill and will fail, over and over, often on purpose, to be quiet when the baby is sleeping. It will be natural for you to cringe when the baby starts to cry in the middle of what you had hoped would be a long nap. I can only offer my empathy for this situation; I know how awful it feels.

However, if you blame the older child for the baby waking, you set yourself up for repeated problems. Instead, decide ahead of time how you want to react when your older child wakes the baby. Focus on the positive. If you emphasize how nice it is to spend time together when the baby is sleeping, and you acknowledge the times when your older child is tiptoeing around quietly, you build good will toward the baby's naps.

Plan Ahead for Situations in which the Baby Gets Hurt

Sooner or later (later if you are lucky), the older sibling is bound to go through a period of wanting to hurt the baby. Often this doesn't rear its ugly head until the baby starts crawling—that's when the little one can get into the older child's play space and wreck his toy creations. Parents naturally feel angry at the older child if he hurts the baby. Our first reaction is often to scold, yell, or punish. Yet, if our goal is to teach the older child empathy and prevent future recurrences, having a prepared reaction to this scenario can help.

If this happens, first, take a deep breath. It is normal. It does not mean anything awful about your older child. He does not hate the baby. He does not have a "problem."

Chick Moorman's course, the "Parent Talk System," offers a great concept for parents called the "Red Light, Green Light" approach. I have used it often and modified it as, the "Red Light, Green Light, Blue Light" approach. You will naturally tell your older child, "You can't hurt the baby." That's the red light. But a red light must be followed by a green light or you will create resentment and problems. If we are driving a car and we only find red lights, we will eventually run them because we are frustrated and there are no other options available to us. Even for adults, there has to be a green light somewhere. A green light would be something like, "If you are frustrated or angry that the baby is taking your toys, you can ask me for help."

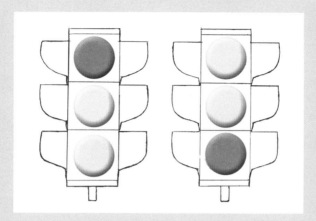

Red Light, Green Light Examples

Other ideas for green lights regarding physical behavior include the following:

BITING:

Red Light: You can't bite the baby.

Green Light: You can bite this cold, wet washcloth if you want. We'll put it right here and whenever you feel like biting, you can come get it. (Hint: Keep it in the refrigerator.)

HITTING:

Red Light: You can't push/hit the baby.

Green Light: If you want, you can always hit the pillow on this couch.

SCREAMING:

Red Light: Screaming at a person is not okay.

Green Light: If you ever feel like screaming, we can go outside and you can scream loudly outdoors. The squirrels don't mind.

Make a plan to talk to your older child at bedtime (or another quiet moment) about how important it is in your family not to hurt each other. This is the blue light—your calm, centered, global approach. Depending on your child's personality and age, you can disguise your blue light in a story. This is surprisingly effective. Starting around age two, you can tell your child bedtime stories including morals you'd like to share. I found it easier to make up stories about wild animals (who just happened to engage in similar behavior to my child) than to find books that conveyed the perfect message. However, there is an impressive array of children's picture books dedicated to helping children through everyday situations. If you are not able to make up stories easily, get to know your local librarian and ask for books with the exact message you are looking for. There is most likely one (or a dozen).

If your child is older or you are short on storytelling time, initiate a simple conversation. In this discussion, you will do your best to focus on the future, not the past. Don't even mention that she pulled the baby's hair that morning. There's no need, as it's done and in the past. As I've mentioned, making your job as protector to include the older child is helpful. I usually start with the phrase, "In this family . . ." Here's a sample for the bedtime talk:

> In this family, we want everyone to feel safe and loved. I love
> you very much and I will always protect you from anyone trying to
> hurt you. If anyone ever tried to hit you, or pinch you, or bite you,
> I would say, 'Stop! That's my little girl! You can't hurt her!' And I
> love Daddy (Mommy) and will always protect him if anyone tries to
> hurt him. And I love Baby and I will always protect him. That's my
> job as your (Mommy) Daddy.

Your child may protest that she knows this already, but it's a gentle way to remind her of the family rules.

I have found there is more attention being paid on how to help siblings get along than there was a generation or two ago. Many good books are available that specifically address sibling issues. I encourage you to be proactive and thoughtful about how to support the relationships between your children. In an ideal world, these relationships will outlast your presence and be a lasting influence on your children and their children as well.

Your Changing Relationship with Your Canine Family Members

Although some tips in this section are applicable to cats (most notably, making any changes you can to your pet's life or routine before your baby is born), most cat owners are able to keep both cat and baby safe without too much extra effort. That is why this section is all about dogs.

Becoming a dog owner is good practice for becoming a parent. Indeed, there are many parallels, especially if you start with a puppy. Puppies need a lot of time and attention, including at night. They are innocent and loving creatures who bring us great joy. Still, sometimes, they make our adult lives difficult. We have to attend to many of their bodily functions that might have seemed unpleasant before we fell in love with the cute little thing. If you are a dog owner, you are already prepared for some realities of life with a baby.

However, you also have new challenges if you bring a human baby home and a dog is already your "baby." Jennifer Shryock, certified dog behavior consultant, thought she knew dogs but found that, "I had lived with dogs, but I had never parented with dogs." Going into this situation with thoughtfulness, rather than being reactive to problems, helps the human and the canine members of the family have a good experience. It's easier to modify behavior with praise (ahead of time) than punishment (afterward).

When I crowd-sourced advice about bringing babies home to pets, by far, the most common recommendation I received was, "Let your pet smell a baby blanket before you bring your baby into the house." Naively, I thought this was great advice, and that the main challenge could be surmounted this easily. If dogs get used to the scent of the baby, then, logically, they would treat the baby the same way they treat other guests who arrive at the house. At first, many dogs are suspicious of new people, but if they are allowed to sniff them, and their owners seem to accept their presence, most dogs will also accept their presence.

When I talked to Cathy Reisfield of "Dependable Dogs," a professional in Ann Arbor, Michigan, who helps dog owners who are also parents, I realized how much more there is to the process. She asks, "What are we expecting if we do this? One sniff does not make a relationship." She goes on to point out, "It's curious in that we don't suggest that other new arrivals to our home send their socks or undergarments ahead for our dogs to sniff ("Oh, you, new people coming for the holidays and staying awhile—send some of your clothing ahead of time!"), but many continue to insist that baby garments and blankets be sent home to dogs." If you do decide to follow this advice, think about how you want your dog to react. You don't want to get the dog excited about the baby's item. Let your dog sniff, get used to the scent, and that's that.

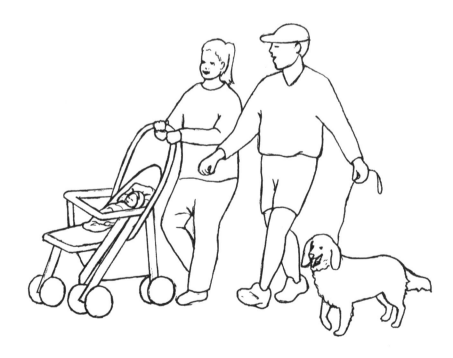

Preparing for the arrival of a baby ahead of time can make a world of difference. There will likely be changes to your dog's routine and additions to your dog's rules. It's better to make those changes while you are pregnant, not after the baby arrives.

For example, if you intend to take your dog for walks while your baby is in a stroller, you should get the stroller early and practice taking it with you on walks. Erlinda, a mother in Fort Wayne, Indiana, found out the hard way that her dog wanted to get into the stroller or pull away from the stroller while they were walking. She ended up having to practice with her dog while her baby was taking naps indoors. Because naptime is so precious, try to make these adjustments ahead of time, if you can. There are more tips from Cathy Reisfield in the sidebar (see pages 130–131).

What to Do After Your Baby Arrives

The two important parts of dog parenting to keep in mind are:

- Maintain a strong connection to your dog
- Monitor the dog–baby relationship so your baby is safe and your dog feels secure

Maintain a Strong Connection As hard as it will be, carve out time to connect with your pet every day. Some new parents can do this from the very beginning. Others find the first two weeks too challenging. Enlist someone to help walk, feed, and play with your dog during this babymoon time. Too often, partners end up on "pet duty" for the first weeks while the new mother rests and breastfeeds.

After the first two weeks, going for a walk is a great activity to help parents engage with their dog. If your baby is in a carrier, you are hands-free and able to walk your dog in a similar fashion to how you did before. Some new parents caution that while carrying their baby, they feel less capable of controlling or protecting their dog when encountering other dogs. This may depend on the size and temperament of your dog as well as your neighborhood experiences.

Dog Preparation and Homecoming

Cathy Reisfield, the creator of the helpful website Dependabledogs.com, offers this quick-reference guide for getting a dog ready for a new baby.

PREPARATION

Preparing your dog *before* the baby's arrival helps increase safety and reduce overall stress. Even the most easygoing dogs, and their owners, benefit from pre-baby preparation. To ready your dog for the changes to come, consider the following:

1. **Assess and improve your dog's basic manners.** If these need work, firm them up before your baby arrives. Useful commands to work on include Polite Greetings, Sit, Down, Wait, and Off (to get off furniture or people when asked).

2. **Practice separation.** Can the dog be away from you behind a gate or in a crate? Teach the dog to relax behind a gate, in another room, on a mat. If you're walking to soothe a fussy baby, an anxious dog underfoot may contribute to your anxiety, in addition to providing a potential tripping hazard.

3. **Assess your dog's anxiety, fear, and aggression toward people.** Ask yourself: What stresses your dog or makes him anxious? How do you know when your dog is stressed? Is he sensitive to loud noises? What about fast movements?

   A little education and knowledge of dog body language goes a very long way. Take time to learn the subtle expressions of dog discomfort and annoyance before you have a mobile baby crawling toward a worried dog. If you have a dog who exhibits fear or aggression toward people, particularly children, it is critical to contact a qualified trainer who can help evaluate the situation and develop a training plan designed to keep everyone safe, while minimizing the dog's anxiety.

4. **Assess how your dog gets attention.** Think about how your dog gets your attention: Barking? Pawing? Stealing items and running off with them? Do these behaviors increase if you ignore them?

   Think about what may happen if you're trying to get the baby to sleep or trying to feed the baby. If you need to alter these behaviors, try to do so now.

5. **Think through new rules that might arise.** Household rules and routines may change when you bring home a baby. Will the dog be permitted in the nursery? If the dog has been sharing your bed, will this need to change as you anticipate being up during the night with a newborn?

As an example, if you have decided your dog will no longer share your bed, don't wait until the day you bring home the baby to make that change. Start to make changes as soon as you can. With all these considerations, don't make assumptions about how your dog will adjust once the baby comes home. Practice. Be patient. Contact a qualified trainer if you need support in addressing these items.

HOMECOMING

Homecoming with your baby should be calm, quiet, and controlled. There is no need for a formal introduction or physical contact between the dog and the baby. When Mom and baby come home for the first time, the dog may be most excited to see Mom and may or may not be curious about the baby.

Mom should greet the dog first without the baby. The baby, in a carrier, should be up on a tabletop or counter, away from the dog, or the baby should be held by another adult.

If the dog is curious about the baby, parents may want to let them meet in a very limited and controlled manner by allowing the dog to sniff the baby's feet—but only under direct adult supervision. If there are concerns about the dog jumping up, consider putting the dog on a leash or having the dog drag a leash. Then you can pick it up or step on it if the dog is over-enthusiastic. Sniffing the baby's feet is a responsible safety precaution. All dogs have teeth. We want to keep those teeth away from the baby's face and head.

When your baby is in a safe place at home, shower your dog with affection when you are able. If relatives or friends visit, make a conscious effort to let your visitors hold the baby while you interact with your dog. Most people are happy to help out in such situations and have such a good reason to hold the baby.

Supervision Reisfield also says that a lack of supervision is the "most common mistake families make." She points out that most of us, even if we conscientiously supervise dog–baby interactions, are uneducated about dog body language and the signs of a problematic interaction. This issue is further compounded by the barrage of distractions in our modern technologically rich life, and by the mere exhaustion of parenting.

Two specific times when it is critically important to be aware of your dog's location and arousal levels are when your baby is sleeping and when you go to the bathroom (or any time you leave the room). Make sure that wherever your baby is put down for a nap is inaccessible to your dog. If you go to the bathroom or leave the room, be certain the dog and the baby are appropriately separated. Reisfield warns that bites can occur, so make it a rule: "Your dog should NEVER have access to your baby without full, awake, adult supervision." She suggests you have a go-to management strategy for separating baby and dog, such as putting the dog behind a baby gate or in a crate. This helps when you have an infant, but "becomes even more important as your baby is more mobile and can move toward your dog and into the dog's personal space."

Make it a point to learn the warning signs that indicate your dog may be experiencing stress. Dogs generally give warnings, through body language and behavior, when they are stressed and likely to lash out in self-protection. Browse websites that can educate you about these signs. Several websites offer photos that compare "stressed" and "calm" dog faces. You may think your dog's open mouth is a sign of happiness; however, there are more physical signals to scan that help you put this sign into perspective. You want to notice, for example, whether your dog's mouth is stretched tightly at the corners of the mouth (a sign of stress) and whether the ears are pinned back (another sign of stress). Websites to browse include http://todaysveterinarypractice.navc.com/.

Finally, if you need immediate support, there is a Dog and Baby Support Hotline at 1-877-247-3407.

Hopefully, with advance planning and attention to your relationship with your dog, your baby will grow up with a wonderful companion. There are so many benefits for your child, including increased empathy and verbal skills, but the most obvious reason to work hard to make your dog and your baby compatible housemates is the expanded love they will learn to give and receive.

Conclusion

Until you bring your first child into your home, there are not many relationships to manage besides the dyad with your partner. You relate to your partner one on one and you relate to your pets, more or less, one on one. When a baby arrives, this changes relationship dynamics dramatically. Now, you are managing your relationship to your partner and your relationship with your child *at the same time*. When siblings are added, the complications increase.

The inherent complications are sometimes difficult to manage, but they are also a source of real joy. Bringing conscious awareness to your relationships, and regularly stepping back from the chaos of the family unit to nurture one-on-one connections, can help everyone feel positive and secure about the whole. Someday, I hope, you will all be together— every person and pet that makes up your unique family—and you will experience that deep satisfaction of looking around and knowing, "This is our family."

THE FOURTH TRIMESTER COMPANION

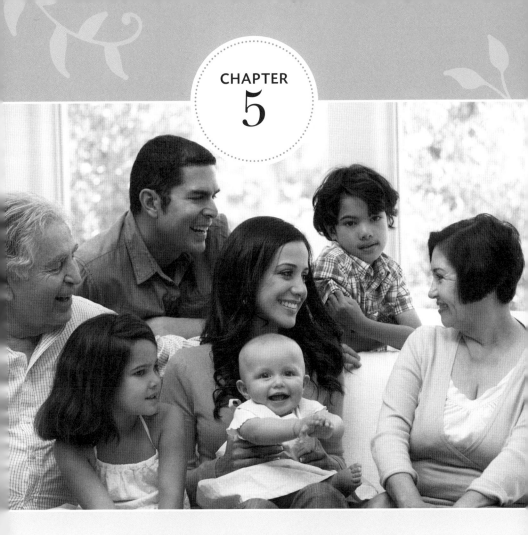

CHAPTER

5

YOUR CHANGING RELATIONSHIPS WITH YOUR PARENTS AND IN-LAWS

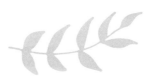

IN THE IMMEDIATE POSTPARTUM, FOURTH TRIMESTER period, I am guided by the belief that a new mother's needs should be realized, accepted, and prioritized. In my vision of the world, laboring women and new mothers are royal queens: whatever they say, goes! This is my wish for all new mothers: that their own parents, in-laws, friends, siblings, and partner are able and willing to support them in whatever way desired for the first three months after the birth. After this fourth trimester, the needs and desires of these other players can begin to fill their proper place in reasonably influencing family decision making. While in practice, this may be impractical, it is a healthy place to start as you plan your postpartum nest.

I do not mean to imply the needs and desires of anyone else are unimportant. However, everyone else can (and should) find ways to get their needs met outside the postpartum nest. Ideally, the new mother should be cocooned with her baby, in a safe and cozy environment, relying on the support of others to keep her "regular world" in motion. She should not be paying bills, raking leaves, or shoveling snow. Even new fathers and other partners, very much a part of the nest, are more able than a breastfeeding, physically recovering mother to sleep through an early morning feeding, take a step outside for fresh air, run to the store, or return to an office job. If the new mother focuses on taking care of the baby, while the partner prioritizes the new mother's care and bond with the baby, the family will be set up for long-term success.

If everyone could set aside their own needs to support new parents exactly as they wished to be supported, this would be a very short chapter. The reality is that nearly all our relationships change when we become mothers. While none of us is usually prepared to handle these adjustments, "forewarned is forearmed," and there *are* ways to smooth these transitions.

If your own parents have died and you won't experience the struggle of navigating this changed dynamic, you may find yourself struggling with some of these issues in relation to your in-laws. (If you are someone who is, or will be, parenting without your own parents, I have written some specific words for you that begin on page 160.)

Your Changing Relationship with Your Parents and Parents-in-Law*: The New Grandparents

As a birth doula who makes prenatal home visits, I often enter a family's home fully prepared to discuss labor and birth. Surprisingly, the discussion of labor is often shunted to a later visit because the discussion about grandparents appears much more pressing. This is especially true when the child to be born will be the first grandchild for one or both sets of grandparents.

It's an Invisible Power Shift

Your relationships with your own parents naturally change when you have a baby. In essence, you take over the very job they've done your entire life: nurturing the next generation. The transformation of your relationship with your family's older generation is usually the most visible challenge of the immediate postpartum period, besides breast-feeding and maintaining your and your baby's health. (Spousal and

---

*Note: *I use the term "parents-in-law" even though some readers may not be married to their partners. I use these "in-law" terms broadly and mean them inclusively for anyone who fits this role in your life.*

partner challenges tend to show up later on.) If you are fortunate enough to discover your relationships with your parents and parents-in-law are nothing but supportive, count your lucky stars and skip ahead in this chapter! Know you are dodging one of the trickiest aspects of new parenthood for many people. Even people with strong, healthy intergenerational relationships find this is a serious adjustment that takes getting used to.

The birth of a baby, especially a first baby, shifts the power dynamic within families dramatically. Unless you grew up in a difficult family, you may not be familiar with "power dynamics" as they apply to your parents. These dynamics are present in every relationship; however, their workings are relatively unconscious for most of us. Up until this point, *you* were the child and your parents were the parents. Although you may have asserted your adulthood in various ways, your parents have mostly continued to be the "official" rule makers. As young adults without children, many of us may have rebelled against some of our parents' rules, but we, most likely, didn't attempt to *make* rules for them.

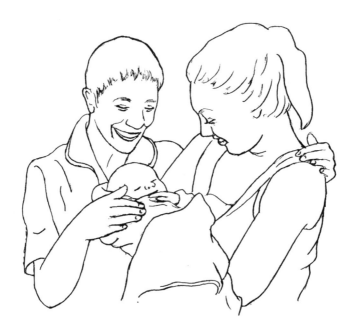

This dynamic changed when you, the child, became a parent. From Day One of this new adventure, you will make rules for and about your child that your parents will have to follow, which is why I call this a power shift.

This does not have to be a negative or melodramatic experience—although, sometimes, it is. Becoming a parent, as well as a grandparent, is a rite of passage. These are critical life transformations that deserve to be recognized with more formality than they are currently regarded in modern Western society. I believe these shifts would be easier to accept, and the losses easier to mourn, if we were more aware of what is happening within and between us.

Grandparents as Respected Elders

Across the globe today (and in the not-so-distant American past), grandparents play a decisive, recognized role in most families. Throughout my travels, the most consistent negative view of Americans I have encountered is that we do not treat our elderly the way we should. The negative aspect of a social obligation to honor elders should be easy enough for Americans to imagine: In many societies, new parents are supposed to bend their wills and wishes to their parents' decisions. Parents have strong influence and even decision-making power over adult children's decisions about who to marry, what profession to enter, and finances. Freedom from this influence does not occur until the older generation dies.

The positives, however, may be harder to see in our fast-paced, technology-driven modern world. Conventional societies view grandparents and elders as reservoirs of experience, knowledge, and tradition. Becoming an elder is an honor, and different rituals and ceremonies help connect elders to babies and define their relationship. Consider the Inuit of northern Canada, for example. When a new baby is born, the elders in the area visit the family and shake the baby's hand to welcome it into the community. They are even held responsible for finding the correct name for the new baby. In the Muslim faith, an elder member of the family is supposed to whisper holy words into babies' ears as the first words they hear.

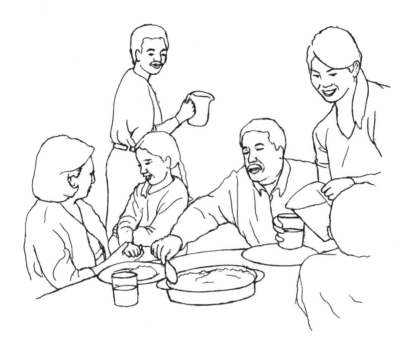

I made a postpartum visit to an Indian-American woman whose baby was eleven days old. Her parents had arrived from India after her baby's birth and were planning to stay for three months. When I was welcomed inside, mouthwatering scents of cardamom and fenugreek came from the kitchen. It was hardly 10:00 in the morning, and multiple pots were already bubbling away on the stove. The young mother had every meal prepared for her by her aunt or mother since she returned home from the hospital, and she always had a mug of herb-steeped water nearby to sip on.

Of course, the new grandparents were excited to hold their grandson, but the first thing this Indian grandmother told me was that her main priority was taking care of her daughter. "We Indians," she said, "believe we should take care of the mother—for forty or forty-five days. We come to wash the mother, wash her hair, wash her body. New mothers are ravenous because they are feeding their babies. You don't want strangers to see the heaps of food she is eating, so close relatives should prepare her food and feed her." Although this might sound like traditional advice, this same grandmother described a successful career in engineering, where she managed mostly male employees. Families who are open to both the traditional and the modern are picking and choosing the best of all worlds.

Across the globe, grandparents provide the majority of childcare that parents cannot provide. In places such as China, India, and Russia, grandparent-provided childcare is a linchpin of the economy. The title of Kelly Yang's 2013 article in *The Atlantic* discussing childcare and working parents in China, says, "In China, It's the Grandparents who 'Lean In.'" That was certainly what I learned in Russia while conducting research there from 2000 to 2001. Grandparents not only provided the bulk of the childcare needs, regardless of social class, they often hosted grandchildren for entire summer vacations at their countryside houses (called dachas). Russian children grew up learning how to collect mushrooms and berries, to fish, and enjoy singing around a campfire with their elders as a matter of course—even if their parents were

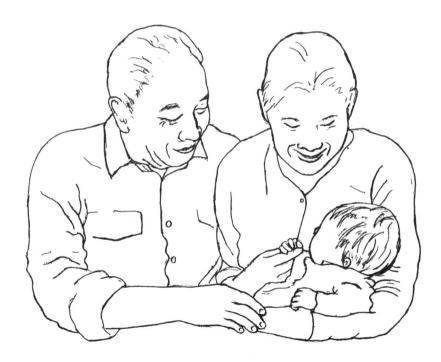

university-educated, urban professionals. The United States, Canada, and Western Europe, by contrast, offer much less value or honor to grandparents, and virtually no traditional rituals.

Becoming a Grandparent in the United States Today: Let Us Acknowledge this Rite of Passage

Take a moment to think about the experience of a baby's birth from a new grandmother's or grandfather's point of view. Surely, becoming a grandparent for the first time is a bittersweet experience in our Western culture.

Grandparents likely experience a mixture of emotions while saying good-bye to things they have valued and cherished. Perhaps they mourn their own youth and the enormous vitality that bringing new life into the world bestows upon new parents. While the new mother confronts a four-to-six-week period of bleeding, her mother may be reminded she is nearing the end of her cycle or that it has ceased. Older parents may be bitter that their time of "rule making" is ending; or, perhaps, they feel relieved. They might be confused about what is expected of them—after all, they are used to thinking of you as young and in need of guidance. Maybe they lived near their own parents, and having felt pressure to submit to their elders far into their own adulthood, unconsciously assume you will follow the same script. In other words, becoming a grandparent for the first time, while undeniably rewarding, can also be emotionally tricky.

More often now, religious organizations acknowledge this transition into "grandparenthood" as a rite of passage. I have been heartened to see many religious communities address the need for more ritual acknowledgment of this experience. For example, in 2007, the Episcopal Church General Convention created a new book of prayers, *Changes: Prayers and Services Honoring Rites of Passage*, which includes blessings for new grandparents. The website Ritualwell.org describes grandparent rituals developed out of the Jewish tradition.

Paradoxically, the reason I am spending so much time on the need for grandparents to be acknowledged is because it helps grandparents and new parents refocus on the deeper, messier, and pressing needs of the new parents. When the needs of grandparents remain hidden and dormant—when nobody recognizes the transition they experience—those needs can, inadvertently, end up center stage. Conversely, when the needs and emotions of new grandparents are acknowledged, proper attention can then be centered on the young, new family.

My advice for new parents is to do whatever they can to make new grandparents feel special, and to openly acknowledge this rite of passage. If you give this some thought during your pregnancy, it will likely help smooth relationship bumps during the postpartum, fourth trimester, period. At the same time, though, protecting the space of a new mother with her baby is paramount. This usually, although not always, involves some creative tension as everyone adjusts to their new roles.

Times Have Changed: Communicating about New Parenting

Most new parents worry about offending their own parents by rejecting their advice on baby care. On the flip side is a concern that the grandparents' outdated philosophy will somehow "ruin" the parents' plans to rear their child the way they see best. It's common that new parenting styles are interpreted as a judgment on the past, but there are ways to navigate this tension and allow everyone to feel included and honored.

The areas of conflict I see most families encounter include differences in opinion (or changes in scientific knowledge) about:

- Breastfeeding
- First foods
- Holding a baby too much, or not enough
- Where a baby sleeps, and how a baby goes to sleep
- Pacifier use and finger sucking

Rather than give you specific advice on each area, I offer ideas I hope you can use in varying situations to help you handle any well-meaning advice with which you disagree. I touch on sleep issues and breast-feeding here, but you will also find more information about these topics in chapters 2 (page 47) and 3 (page 69).

Ask about Their Experiences and Be a Good Listener!

Many women grow up hearing stories about their mother's pregnancy, birthing, and breastfeeding experiences, but will likely ask for more

Generational Conflict and Resolution Stories

DIALOGUE

Jordan: *I got really caught up in trying to get my newborn to sleep in her bassinet because my nana, mum, and mother-in-law said I should. It was stressful for us all and, once I stopped trying to make her sleep there, we all slept one hundred times better! I was a first-time mum, and my partner and I lived three hours away from our family, so I had no local support. I had read the SIDS guidelines prior to giving birth, and thought I was doing something wrong because she never wanted to stay asleep in the bassinet. I remember my nana saying, "She MUST sleep in her own bed!" Looking back now, it's just an old-school mentality; my dad said I was put in a cot in my own room the night we got home from hospital.*

It felt natural to let her sleep on my chest during the day and by my side at night. I don't remember if there was a particular reason I stopped trying with the bassinet, but, shortly after, we sold her cot and now, at almost two, she sleeps in a double bed.

An aunt told me it wasn't good for our relationship to have our daughter in the bed. I told her the bed wasn't the only place we could have sex, and that more sleep for everyone means happier parents!

If we have another baby, we will co-sleep. Now, I also know the safe bed-sharing guidelines, and that SIDS risk is actually reduced if you are a breastfeeding mother!

Fae: *My grandmother told me I needed to have bottles and formula ready, as she was unable to breastfeed my mother (and then went into detail of a breast black with mastitis). That my mother couldn't breast-feed, nor my aunty. That I had such a flat chest that I, too, wouldn't be able to breastfeed. Little did she know I took that as a challenge, and went on to exclusively breastfeed all five of my kids for two years or more each. Take that, Negative Nelly Grandma!*

Serena: *I have faced pressure from my parents, but also my grand-parents. I find my grandmother the most difficult, as things were so different when she had babies. She told me a story the other day about how she had to stop breastfeeding at six weeks as both my dad and aunty got pimples on their face because her "milk was too rich" for them. That was what she was told back then, and what she believes is true. It's hard to convince someone that something she has believed for sixty years isn't true!*

Daphne: *Everyone has an opinion regarding babies and children—even those who don't have children! Opinions are okay, but having one doesn't mean it's what's right. I've always listened politely to others' advice and opinions, but have always had the mentality: "My baby, my rules." Instead of arguing, I would often just smile and nod, then do my own thing! My husband and I have never felt the need to justify or explain our parenting choices. Now that we have three children, no one really gives me their opinion anymore.*

details once they are expecting their first child. I encourage you to explore your mother's (and, if you can, your grandmothers') experiences and see how they fit within their historical era. It can also be useful to ask direct questions about their early parenting experiences with their own relatives. Did they feel supported? Where were areas of conflict? If you can, engage with genuine curiosity about how early parenting felt for them. Many women find these conversations alone are enough to validate everyone's feelings and create a solid base of mutual understanding.

Smile When They Give Advice and Do What You Want Anyway

Remember, you do not have to convince anyone you are right in order to parent the way you'd like. It is absolutely okay if someone disagrees with you. You do not have to fight about it. If you know there are areas of disagreement, tell yourself just to smile, nod, and refuse to argue whenever the topic arises.

This will happen naturally as you become a more experienced parent. One mother, Kelly Bolan, recalls, "Wow! All the struggles I felt with my first. Everything was an issue: breastfeeding, co-sleeping, baby-wearing. I felt a huge push against me. On to baby number three and I could give a Crayola about what anyone else thinks!"

You do not have to wait until you have three children to put this advice to work for you!

Practice Ahead of Time and Practice Out Loud

I've discovered that rehearsing something difficult in my life helps prepare me for the actual moment. For example, if you know you will encounter relatives with strong, dissenting opinions, ask a friend to role-play what it might be like to hear their advice. You can practice smiling, nodding, and changing the topic. I did this recently with a pregnant client. Her mother was firmly against the baby sleeping in the same room (in a co-sleeper) with her. In my role-play, I exaggerated how awful this judgmental mother might be, and my client practiced deflecting her unwanted advice. We ended up laughing so much, my sides hurt and tears were coming out of my eyes! She texted me about two weeks after her baby was born to tell me that whenever her mother makes a comment about how inappropriate it is to sleep near her baby, she remembers our hysterical laughter together, and is able to smile and move on without getting upset.

Go to a Mothering Support Group with Like-Minded New Mothers

If you are lucky enough to live in the same town you grew up in, and you have cousins, siblings, or close friends with babies, you may already have a built-in support group of mothers. Unfortunately, this is not the case for most mothers I meet.

In my case, I gave birth to each of my three children in different places: New York City, Toronto, and Ann Arbor, Michigan. In each of these cities, I had to begin at square one to find like-minded friends. When I had my third baby, I wasn't sure I needed to do this anymore. After all, I was already close to the parents of my older children's friends. However, I was pleasantly surprised at how useful it was to be in a mom–baby support group and connect with other women navigating the same things I was: getting a baby to sleep, breastmilk leakage in the grocery store, blow-out diaper changes on car trips. I needed their compassion and understanding for my sanity. My other friends with older children had moved on from these baby-life concerns.

Ask Your Partner to Answer for Both of You and Present a United Front

This advice does not work for everyone for the obvious reason that not everyone has a partner, nor are partners always on the same page about parenting. However, if you have a partner and you're both on the same page, it can be effective to appoint the one who has not just endured labor and delivery (and who is not dealing with engorged breasts) to respond to parenting advice. Danielle, who lives in Australia, shares one of her encounters with unsolicited advice:

People always have opinions. We plan to keep our preschool-age children home, and my husband's aunt kept talking about how good preschool would be for our son. I tried to be polite, but I guess I wasn't firm enough! She eventually brought it up to my husband, and he very firmly told her we weren't sending him to preschool, and described all the activities he does at home and with other kids—and she hasn't mentioned it since. I think if hubby can field some of the advice it may make it easier on new parents. I think once people realize you are both on the same page, they tend to leave you alone.

A united front can make someone giving unwanted advice realize the decision has already been made and their role is not that of the decision maker.

Imagine How a "Perfect Parent" Would React

You probably already realize your parents are not perfect. However, imagining what "the perfect parent" would do in any given situation can help you find more space for your own ideas. I find it helps me remember that my parents do not *have* to react the way they do. They have choices—and so do I.

Chloe, a friend who lives in Seattle, was deeply saddened when her mother decided to go on a four-month-long trip that began two weeks after her second baby was born. Her mother had been a great help to her in the fourth trimester after her first baby, and she had hoped her mother would be there to support her again. Although Chloe expressed her wish that her mother postpone her trip, she still left on schedule. In this situation, it was very clear what a "perfect parent" would have done: respect her daughter's request, and stay home to help for several weeks.

In other cases, it's not immediately clear what "perfect parents" would do. Still, the thought experiment can be helpful. My doula partner, Martha Hollis, and I once had a conversation with a couple expecting their first baby around Christmas. At first, they were excited because they had managed, for the first time ever, to beg off traveling to their hometown for the holidays. Their due date of January 1 was an easy excuse that all their relatives accepted as a valid reason to not be hours away from home. They would celebrate Christmas in their own home for the first time! Unfortunately, no sooner had this victory occurred when each set of parents made plans to visit the week following Christmas. The father-to-be had two weeks off work for the holiday, and the couple had been looking forward to spending this time together before their baby arrived. Now it would be broken up by visits from both sets of parents and, instead of relaxed snuggling and bonding, they foresaw the expectations of hosting.

As we talked with this couple, we told them our idea of the "hypothetical perfect parent" and what that ideal would look like.

HYPOTHETICAL PERFECT PARENTS

☑ Do not get offended when their grown children take time alone or away from them. They respect that their adult children need privacy and space.

☑ Do not keep tabs on who is invited and who is left out of anything. They trust the new parents to decide how and when to include relatives and friends.

☑ Offer to help whenever they can, but are open to their adult children's requests that their help come in a different form than originally offered.

☑ Offer advice when asked, but say nothing if not asked.

☑ Are willing to learn how the parents do things instead of rigidly insisting their own way is better.

☑ Remember to pamper and care for the new parents as much as the new baby.

Together, we brainstormed the following ideas regarding their current situation: "Hypothetical perfect parents" would have called to say they were very sad about not seeing us for Christmas, that they couldn't really imagine a holiday season without us for at least a short visit, and that they wanted to come visit. However, they would go on to explain, they did not want to intrude, so they would be happy to consider plans that might work for everyone. Ideas might include staying at a hotel (instead of at the couple's home) and coming for a one-afternoon visit instead of overnight. Still, they would understand and not be offended if the couple expressed a desire to have their own time and space before the baby's arrival.

This imagination exercise did not solve the problem; however, it did lead to a discussion of alternative endings. Just because their parents made plans without asking permission first, does not mean the couple must go along with the plan. They have the ability, and responsibility to themselves, to suggest alternatives more palatable to them. I've found that imagining the "hypothetical perfect parent" and brainstorming what that parent might do, has helped people feel differently about their situations and their power in them. This exercise not only uncovered alternative ways their parents *could have acted*, it revealed more options for the couple, too.

Many of us get caught up in reacting to our own parents and parents-in-law within the paradigm we've always lived in. Up to this point, it likely was one of very few options, as the older generation held some invisible power that allowed them to make rules and define situations as they saw best. Now, you are no longer the "child" in these scenarios. You are a parent as well, and your decisions will shape the lives and experiences of your own children. Concentrate on what is right for you and your family, and model the kind of compassionate person you'd like your children to be when they grow up.

Someday, when your child is an adult and asks for time or space, hopefully, you will cheerfully allow them what's needed without a guilt trip. Similarly, if you have the mental and emotional capacity to give the new grandparents some of what they want and need, I encourage you to do so. Stretching yourself to meet their needs is an act of love, but *only* if it does not impinge on your ability to rest and recover, breastfeed and bond, and find mental peace in the early days of this fourth trimester.

Breastfeeding Challenges with Parents or Parents-in-Law

If your parents and grandparents were born in the United States, they likely were formula-fed, even if their mothers started off breastfeeding. Some mothers bucked this trend, but, statistically, formula-feeding dominated from the 1960s until the 1980s. If mothers did breastfeed, they likely received breastfeeding advice based on the science of formula-feeding, which recommended that babies be fed on a schedule (every three to four hours) and would not need feedings in between those scheduled times.

Millions of Americans are alive and healthy today who were formula- or schedule-fed as babies. It makes sense that our mothers and grandmothers see no reason to change what worked for them.

There are two common areas of potential conflict surrounding breastfeeding that may come up in the early postpartum period, and a third area you can, hopefully, fend off until later. The first potential conflict regards breastfeeding itself. Your parents or parents-in-law might question the need to breastfeed your baby at all, especially if you have difficulty. A second conflict may arise concerning modesty (or a lack thereof). In the first few weeks, and even months, mothers and babies are just getting the hang of breastfeeding, and it can indeed be a messy and revealing affair. Thirdly, you may encounter differences of opinion about how long you should breastfeed your child, but this should not be a pressing conflict in the early weeks.

In the last generation, much more in-depth research has been conducted on breastfeeding and formula-feeding. The preponderance of evidence now supports the claim that breastmilk is the best food for infants, and creates a lifelong foundation for the child's health. More hospitals are using donor milk for NICU babies when needed, because of the proven health benefits. In addition, breastfeeding dramatically reduces the mother's risk of breast cancer—the longer she breastfeeds, the lower her risk becomes. I know breastfeeding is rarely impossible, yet for those situations I am as grateful as anyone that science has produced formula. Still, whenever possible, breast is clearly best.

Most of the time, new grandparents will not argue too much about this—until breastfeeding challenges arise. Then, exactly when a new mother most needs support and encouragement, she might hear advice like, "I bottle-fed you, and you turned out fine!" or "I couldn't produce milk either! It's nothing to be ashamed of." If breastfeeding is working well for you, most advice I've provided previously will be sufficient to stay your course and maintain a positive relationship with your parents and parents-in-law. However, if you experience challenges with breastfeeding, you may benefit from reading further.

When There Are Breastfeeding Challenges

If you struggle in any way with breastfeeding, I urge you to call in support. Reach out to lactation consultants, a postpartum doula, or a close friend with breastfeeding experience. Many lactation consultants will come to your house to help you in the first two weeks. This is expensive, but worth every penny if it helps you continue your breastfeeding journey. LaKesha, mother of two and a La Leche League (LLL) leader, points out that after the first two weeks, it is easier for new mothers to leave the house and go to mom–baby groups and LLL meetings. In those places, you can receive free (or low-cost) support and encouragement. So, when you look at the price of a lactation consultant home visit, remember it is a temporary cost, and that you will, likely, be able to access free or low-cost help very soon if the struggle continues.

Janice, a mother in Orlando, Florida, inadvertently discovered that inviting her birth doula to her house while her parents were visiting helped her find her own voice. Her doula was giving breastfeeding tips during a routine postpartum visit and had assumed everyone present was supportive of Janice's decision to breastfeed. In fact, her mother had been very worried that Janice was not making enough milk and that the baby needed supplementation.

Janice's doula chattered about babies and weight loss and gain, just rattling off facts probably not available to Janice's mother when she had her own babies. Janice wrote to her doula later saying, "I can't thank you enough for all the things you said about how good breastfeeding is. My mom is now a complete convert and is telling all her friends about it. I think she is wishing she had stuck to it more when we were little."

If you do not have a postpartum doula, but you have a female friend who is supportive and understanding of breastfeeding, invite her over to help you. She may not have all the skills of a lactation consultant, but she can bolster your self-confidence in front of your relatives and remind you of what *you* want for *your* baby.

Advice on Sleeping

As you know from earlier chapters, I am an advocate of new parents getting sleep however works best for them. I see a *mother's* sleep as the real issue, not the baby's sleep! Whatever a new mother needs to do to get enough sleep to function well is what she should do. That said, most of the time I work with families either planning some version of co-sleeping, or planning to sleep separately, but eventually ending up sharing their room or bed. Any kind of co-sleeping tends to run counter to the strong cultural messages we receive about infant sleep—and the messages your mother and grandmother likely received. However, if the situation is reversed (your parents can't understand why you are using a crib), you are just as in need of support.

Everyone asks how your baby is sleeping. They say, "How cute! How adorable! How does she sleep?" Then people give loads of unsolicited advice or tell horror stories about baby sleep. This is hard enough, but when it is your parents or parents-in-law giving you advice, it can feel like a strong, uphill battle to try out your own ideas. Sleep, unlike infant feeding, can usually be done out of view. Of course, if your parents live with you or visit for an extended period, this can be trickier.

My experience with new parents convinces me that part of what new parents need is more confidence to stand up for themselves. Ask yourself whether the person giving you advice about sleep is going to *lose any sleep* tonight by following his or her own advice. If not, please take this as a signed permission slip to ignore the opinions and do what feels right to you.

Your parents or parents-in-law, if they oppose bed-sharing or co-sleeping, likely do so because they believe some old-fashioned ideas such as "beds are only for marriage partners," or "babies will become spoiled if you answer their cries at night," or "babies will never learn how to sleep through the night if you keep answering them at night." Younger people who oppose co-sleeping, such as your pediatrician or close friends, are more likely to cite SIDS as the reason. Please read chapter 2 (see page 47) for more specific information about family sleep and the reasons babies wake and sleep the way they do. In this chapter, be sure to read the sidebars (pages 144–145) from women who successfully navigated conflict with the older generation when caring for a baby.

The message offered by many mothers who have been there before you is, be confident in your choices—and in your right to make your own choices—right now. If you have more children, you will likely develop that assurance over time. You will learn what works for you, and for your children. However, there is no reason not to cultivate self-confidence from the beginning, with your first child. If something doesn't feel right, and you suspect you are doing something because it makes someone else happy, change what you are doing. You are the parent!

A Short History of Birth and Parenting

How your Great-Grandmother, Grandmother, and Mother might have been Born and Raised

Understanding some history of birth and parenting in the Western world is helpful for many new parents today. You may feel more empathy for your relatives if you see the experiences of your mother, aunts, grandmothers, and great-grandmothers within their generational context. These are the women we naturally turn to for advice and help. Were their experiences part of the mainstream, or were they born into countercultural families?

If we are lucky, they parented in ways we appreciate and want to emulate. Some of us, on the other hand, so dislike the way we were raised that we vow to do the exact opposite of anything our parents did. Most of us fall somewhere in the middle.

1950 to 60s

Your female ancestor born during this period was probably born in a hospital (possibly part of the first generation in her family to be born there), and though she was more likely to have been bottle-fed than breastfed, there was also a very good chance she may have been breastfed in the early 1950s. Her father was extremely unlikely to have attended her birth.

In the 1950s, virtually all American babies were born in hospitals. Many women, especially poor women, gave birth without any drugs, but many were given the so-called "Twilight Sleep" drugs. They felt the pain of childbirth, but later had no memories of it. Fathers and other support people were not welcome in the birthing room.

Women were exhorted to be "perfect" housewives after WWII, an age that revered science. America's ability to build and use an atomic bomb was considered a positive example of the power of science. Companies touted all kinds of fancy-sounding products, such as Lysol and Colgate, that seemed better than the old, more natural products that reminded everyone of living on farms (vinegar and baking soda, for example). It made sense that, during this era, many people—doctors and new mothers alike—thought science had improved on the messy process of breastfeeding with the development of formula. Breastfeeding became associated with being poor and underprivileged. In the early 1950s, white mothers breastfed their babies for three months or longer only 28 percent of the time. That means virtually three-quarters of white babies were bottle-fed! Black mothers breastfed more often in the 1950s but, by the 1970s, the switch to formula was virtually complete for all families.

The "scientific" rationale of the post-war era encompassed far more than *what* the baby was supposed to eat. It also prescribed how often the baby should eat, how babies should sleep, and how parents and babies should interact. Parents were told it was best to feed babies on schedules, let babies cry it out to learn to fall asleep independently, give babies lots of time on flat surfaces so their spines would grow straight, and separate the adults from the children at night. Not only was this considered the right and proper way to care for infants, it

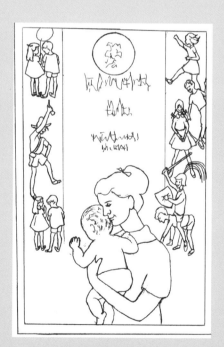

THE FOURTH TRIMESTER COMPANION

was also patriotic and "American." A popular book, written by Walter Sackett in 1962, forbade nighttime feedings and picking up babies when they cried. Sackett wrote, "If we teach our offspring to expect everything to be provided on demand, we must admit the possibility that we are sowing the seeds of socialism." Bucking medical advice was equated with being anti-American.

1970 through the Mid-1980s

If your ancestor was born under Twilight Sleep and/or by cesarean section, and was formula-fed, she experienced the babyhood most common to babies in America during this time. Her father, likely, did not attend her birth. If she were born naturally and breastfed, it likely meant her mother was either quite poor, quite rural, and/or quite determined.

Birthing and parenting had become so "scientific" by the 1970s and 1980s it is no wonder a backlash flourished. Although "Lamaze" became a household term as women began to question the medical model of birth, the natural birth movement was not large or mainstream in this time period. By the late 1970s, fathers were welcomed in birth rooms, in part because women were no longer under the influence of Twilight Sleep drugs. Now, epidurals had emerged as the drug of choice for childbirth. Midwives (hospital and homebirth midwives) emerged from the shadows and became increasingly organized, though not wholly visible to the mainstream.

Breastfeeding was at an all-time low in the early 1970s. In 1971, white mothers breastfed their babies for three months or more only 8 percent of the time, and black mothers only 2 percent. That means that 92 to 98 percent of babies were formula-fed! Your mother or grandmother, if she were a baby in the United States at this time, was *very likely* formula-fed. The breastfeeding tradition, a link from one generation to the next that had been ongoing for hundreds of thousands of years, was broken that quickly.

Dr. Spock's advice, the natural birth movement, and La Leche League (all born in the post-WWII era, but reaching the masses more fully in the 1970s) helped some women give birth and parent in less rigidly programmed ways. However, the philosophies of spoiling babies with too much holding, and feeding babies on a clock, were still dominant in this era.

Late 1980s through 1990s

Your ancestor had a one-in-four chance of being born by cesarean, and was probably born while her mother received an epidural for pain relief. Her father was likely at her birth. She was also more likely to have been breastfed than her own mother, especially in the first few days of life, although she was still statistically much more likely to have been formula-fed than breastfed in the first months. Your ancestor may have been born to a mother who actively sought out midwifery and/or doula care, and a natural birth experience.

The natural birth movement was vocal and more mainstream during this period. At the same time, birth became more medicalized than ever. More women experienced cesareans than ever before in human history. According to the CDC, by 2000, the cesarean rate had reached nearly one-fourth of all U.S. births. (It is now even higher, at 32 percent of all U.S. births). The split between those who advocated for and believed in "natural birth," and advocates of "medicalized birth," was becoming more visible and fractious. At the same time, as more women experienced medical interventions in their labors, more women were hiring midwives and doulas than ever before. Midwifery practices grew rapidly at hospitals across the United States, and doulas emerged as an official profession.

Lessons to Learn

I believe the following central ideas from this short history are helpful to remember:

1. Americans today are one generation apart from an almost-total reliance on formula.

No wonder many of us have breastfeeding challenges! The incredibly high rates of bottle-feeding in the early 1970s meant an entire generation, more or less, never interacted with breastfeeding women and babies. Smaller family sizes mean, even if your mother was one of those in the 1980s or '90s who returned to breastfeeding, you probably do not remember *seeing* your mother breastfeed a sibling.

2. Your parents likely made choices (about baby sleep, infant feeding, etc.), based on philosophies considered best choices at the time.

Your parents may not have read anything current about the changes in expert recommendations since they had young children, so these new ideas may sound like a bunch of crazy Millennial talk to them. I know of one young mother who, literally, pulled a book off her mother's shelf (it had been sitting there for twenty-eight years) and sat down with her to compare the old advice to the new advice. She describes the effect it had:

> When I told my mother about our plans to co-sleep and breastfeed for more than three months, she thought I was being a liberal hippie and that I would, in her words, "ruin" my child. I showed her the scientific evidence about breastfeeding and found the places in her old book that have now been proven wrong. She didn't really seem to believe me at first, but, later, I heard her telling her sister that maybe I grew up with so many allergies because of formula.
> She never said she thought I was right, but I was able to ignore her comments about being a hippie after that.

Your parents have a stake in believing that *you* turned out all right. That knowledge (that you turned out all right despite their "mistakes") is actually more helpful to you than you might think. Human babies are able to survive—and go on to thrive—in an amazing variety of situations. Humans are incredibly adaptable, and the mistakes you make (I operate under the assumption that making mistakes is an unavoidable fact of parenting), *may* scar your child for life, but they will also shape your child into a unique, interesting adult.

You will probably look back on your own early parenting efforts and laugh at yourself. So if you can take yourself a little less seriously now, go ahead and do it!

Parenting without Your Own Parent(s)

When you have a baby after your parents have already died, you may experience things very differently in the postpartum period than your peers. In fact, you are likely to have many differences, even from your partner whose parents are still living. You know this intuitively, but you may not realize how common your feelings and behavior are among other parentless parents.

In your case, preparing for parenthood involves preparing for these experiences. I include thoughts, too, that others have shared about this transition.

1. Be prepared for deep sadness and unanswered questions.

As you navigate early parenting, there will surely be 101 things you would have casually asked your own parents. These are questions most of us never ask when we are teenagers or young adults. After all, in what context would we ask our mother whether she leaked milk constantly for weeks after her milk came in? Samantha, whose mother died only the year before she got pregnant, says, "It hits me daily. All the times I think of just calling her and asking a question, and then remembering all over again I can't do that. Just yesterday, Jared (her three-month-old) finally got his thumb in his mouth by himself, on purpose. He was so happy! Did I suck my thumb? I don't think so. But now I'll never know for sure."

2. You might feel jealous of your partner's parents.

If you're wishing your children could get to know your own parent(s), but never will, it makes sense you may feel some jealousy toward the relationships your in-laws are able to create with their grandchildren. Allison Gilbert, author of *Parentless Parents: How the Loss of Our Mothers and Fathers Impacts the Way We Raise Our Own Children*, relates this about her own experience:

Sometimes just the physical presence of Mark's parents—and the disproportionate representation of their interests and values—have the potential to marginalize what I bring to the parenting table.

The widespread ripple effects are easy to imagine. You might feel self-conscious hanging Christmas stockings if your spouse (and her entire family) celebrates Chanukah. If your parents believed kids shouldn't watch a lot of TV and your in-laws have the television on every time your children visit, you may feel like you're swimming upstream—especially if your partner follows his parents' example at home.

Holidays, as Gilbert notes, are times when this imbalance is felt acutely. You likely miss your own parent(s) more during holidays, and are also aware of what your children are missing.

3. You might fear that you will die early.

Becoming a parent makes us all more aware of life's fragility and causes us to worry, at least a little, about what will happen if we die before our children grow up. If you have experienced the premature death of a parent, this fear may be more palpable for you. Gilbert relates the following anecdotes:

One mom told me that because her in-laws are alive, she and her husband often approach parenting from very different perspectives. "That's been a huge issue for us. He's not trained to think of the worst-case scenario. Whereas, when I see a situation, my mind goes immediately to what could happen." She says her husband has called her "paranoid" and "neurotic."

Another mom reflected that she often pushes her children to be far more independent than her husband likes. "I actually parent with the idea that I could be gone tomorrow," she said.

Although statistically unlikely, because you have already experienced the reality of an early parent death, you are more likely to be aware of this possibility than your friends or your partner.

4. You might find more freedom than other parents.

Even though no one would wish for or welcome the early death of a parent, some individuals to whom this has happened find they feel more liberated than their peers to parent the way they desire. Jeanne Safer, a psychotherapist in New York, has written about the hidden "death benefits" of losing a parent. She finds that many adults can make changes in their lives—after losing a parent—that they were unable to make before.

Support groups for mothers who have lost their own mothers, inspired by Hope Edelman, author of *Motherless Mothers: How Losing a Mother Shapes the Mother You Become*, exist across the world. As with so much in life, it can help, more than you imagine, to know others have felt like you do now. If there is not a face-to-face support group in your area, look online or read one of the two books mentioned in this chapter. Hope Edelman's website, Hopeedelman.com, lists support groups for mothers who have lost their mothers.

Conclusion

"It takes a village" sounds trite; however, it is true. Parenting is not ever an independent task, even though for days and weeks at a time it can seem that way. Hopefully, your parents and, if you have a partner, your partner's parents are part of your village. Even if you lean on other friends or family members for most of your support, grandparents offer an important connection to the past for your children.

Becoming a parent fundamentally changes your relationship with your family elders. You step into a new role, and so do they. This happens even if your parents are no longer alive, because you start to see and understand your own childhood from a new perspective—a parent's perspective. Now that you are nurturing a little one, I urge you to seek out nurturing for yourself ("mothering for the mother" as we doulas call it) from your real parents or from parent figures in your life. The village should nurture everyone.

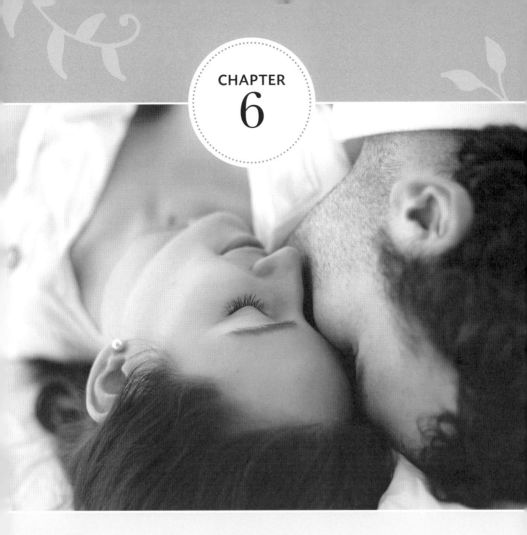

CHAPTER
6

YOUR
SEXUALITY

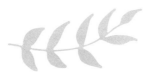

N O ONE TALKS ABOUT THE SEX LIFE OF NEW PARENTS. Most of us expect to return to our pre-pregnancy sex life by six weeks or so after our babies are born. This is what we are led to believe by many birth books and practitioners, yet this expectation is not realistic—and, unfortunately, few discuss this topic openly.

Deep, meaningful conversations considering the nuances of real-life sexual relationships are minimal; even our exposure to sex in the media is fanciful and misleading, at best. This leaves most people struggling in silence by themselves. Fortunately, it doesn't have to be this way.

I have struggled with my own sexuality in the wake of becoming a mother. I'm certain I would have benefitted from some advice, and a few reality checks, when my children were small. I feel privileged to have had the opportunity to break this wall of silence with several hundred women over the years, during interviews and within mother–baby groups. New mothers everywhere struggle to make sense of their bodies and their intimate relationships after giving birth. You are not alone.

The truth is that postpartum sex is a continuation of your existing sex life. Friends, family, and medical professionals may assume you haven't had

The truth is that postpartum sex is a continuation of your existing sex life.

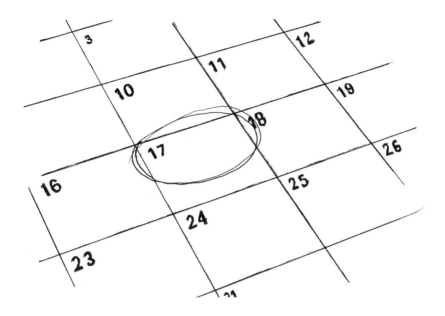

sex in a *long* time, as if pregnancy and sex were incompatible. Although pregnancy does slow down a sex life for some couples, for other couples pregnancy it is a time of great sexual exploration. Even so, birth has a way of changing the sexual dynamic, even if you were fully enjoying yourselves just a few days or weeks ago.

Some challenges will naturally present themselves, considering the physical experiences of labor, delivery, and lactation. However, many challenges to a having a regular, enjoyable sex life after birthing a baby have to do with *living with a baby*. Sometimes, it's the partner who doesn't yet feel ready to resume an active, regular sex life, adjusting to new family roles and the existence of the baby. This interruption that babies bring to a sexual relationship was made clear to me when I interviewed several families who had adopted their infants. These couples described many of the same challenges birth parents face.

Although some couples are able to pick up right where they left off without any trouble (and may not need this section of the book at all), most couples learn there is an adjustment period. It is absolutely normal if your libido, feelings about yourself and your partner, and your sex life go through a fine-tuning period. Here are some thoughts about post-partum sex I have culled from research, interviews, and online anonymous surveys I conducted about this topic.

Have Realistic Expectations

The truth is that 38 percent of us have sexual difficulties even before we have babies, and 83 percent of us are not having the same kind of sex life we're used to for up to *three months* or even *six months* (64 percent) after having a baby. In other words, it is *normal* to have a very different kind of sex life for a long time after our babies are born. It is unusual to return to an easy, effortless sex life within six months postpartum.

Medical professionals, some therapists, and certainly our main-stream media, can easily pathologize our sex lives when they don't fit a pre-existing ideal. In 2000, researchers in the *British Journal of Obstetrics and Gynecology* reported those same statistics I just quoted, but in a very different way. They write, "Sexual morbidity increased significantly after the birth: in the first three months after delivery 83 percent of women experienced sexual problems, declining to 64 percent at six months, although not reaching pre-pregnancy levels of 38 percent." What appears to be very *normal*, that is to have a disrupted, changed sex life in the first six months after having a baby, is pathologized as "sexual morbidity" here. I think it is important for us to talk more openly about the realities of postpartum life, including postpartum sex, so we can better see what the range of "normal" is, and appreciate what is happening without worry.

Don't be fooled by the sex surveys you read in magazines—even some of the more respected magazines. Any time they provide a survey about sex, they attract a certain kind of response. While researching this chapter, I was dismayed at how many seemingly trustworthy "studies" reported that postpartum couples have sex several times a week or more. It did not take much poking around to realize anonymous self-reporting magazine studies clearly attract respondents who have active sex lives or want to appear to have active sex lives. The research conducted by medical and social science researchers, who draw participants from among populations that more closely resemble the general population, reveals a more complex story (and less active sex lives).

We can be very clear about this: *The time it takes to return to sex varies greatly, but will usually be longer than you expect.* Many people assume that the six-week mark is a magical date because there is usually a checkup at six weeks with a doctor or midwife, who will typically give you the go ahead. Indeed, one of the topics of conversation at this checkup is

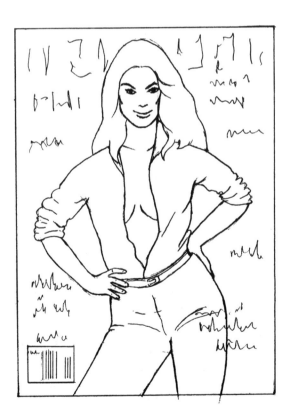

supposed to be birth control and, yes, the medical professional will examine the perineal area and abdomen for healing. However, this does not mean that a magic date has arrived. Do not think for a moment that most people have sex sometime around the six-week mark. Some do—but many, many, *many* do not. My surveys, which corroborate the information I've gathered over the years from mom–baby groups, indicate about 20 percent of couples have their first sexual encounter around the six-week mark. About 26 percent engage even earlier (between two and five weeks postpartum). But the majority of couples (54 percent) wait longer than six weeks, and more than 12 percent wait six months or longer.

The First Time Is Often an Experiment

The first time you have sex after having a baby is more of a "check in" than an act of passion, and it may continue this way for a while.

A woman often wonders what sex will feel like after having a baby, even if she gave birth by cesarean. Many things feel different in her body and it's not clear to her ahead of time how these new sensations will affect sex. Lactating women are likely experiencing leaking and spraying as part of their everyday lives, and may worry about how it will affect the sexual experience. A woman who might have previously relied on nipple stimulation to help reach arousal, may worry that her nipples are too sore from her baby's mouth to be played with as they were in the past. Fernanda, mother of two in Eugene, Oregon, said she found that her nipples felt as though they "belonged" to her baby, so breast foreplay was put to the side for a while. Still, you don't know your answers to any of these questions until you try.

Women whose birthing experience was difficult or traumatic may feel triggered by the idea or experience of introducing anything into her vagina. For example, Anna-Rosa, a mother who planned a natural birth but gave birth by cesarean, found herself crying uncontrollably the first time she had sex with her husband postpartum. She thinks it was a release of some unrealized sadness she harbored about her baby *not* emerging from her vagina. Luckily, her husband understood, and the next times felt less emotional for her.

If you approach the first time—and, realistically, the first five or six times—as experiments, you are less likely to be disappointed. These are occasions for you and your partner to figure out what will work for you; these are definitely not opportunities to measure or define your sexual success.

The Second Time May Be a Long Way Off

Your second attempt at having sex may not follow closely on the heels of the first. About 40 percent of women I surveyed report that their second sex act occurred within two weeks of the first. Yet, the other 60 percent say it took them longer than two weeks to return to this intimacy.

There are plenty of reasons for this. One reason might be that a couple normally takes time between sexual encounters. David Schnarch, Ph.D., studied more than 20,000 couples and found that only a quarter of them have sex once a week on average. Far more commonly reported in his study was the occurrence of sex once or twice a month.

Of course, another reason may well be physical discomfort. If the first attempt reveals to the postpartum mother that sex can be painful in some way, it is a likely reason to delay the next sexual engagement. If having sex is painful, and visiting the doctor is logistically difficult as a new mother, she might wait it out and hope time heals the problem. It can be demoralizing to find out there is pain. After such enormous physical experiences as pregnancy, labor, delivery, and lactation naturally are (especially if any of those did not go as planned), it can be disheartening to discover sex has become yet another physical issue that must be dealt with. Isn't it supposed to be fun and relaxing, and not some chore on a to-do list? With grace and patience, your return to intimacy can be a sweet and gentle experience. Following, I've included for you some tips on handling the pain.

You May Both Need Reassurance This section is helpful to share with your partner. Women are often anxious and fretful about how their partner will see them now. Indeed, they need reassurance, but part of that need is not wanting to ask for it.

At the same time, the partner is likely to need and want reassurance, as well, to know that she is still desirable, and that the birth mother is not so wrapped up in the infant there is no room left for their intimate sexual bond.

The unfortunate news for partners is that a new mother is in no position to offer this reassurance. She will be able to do this better once the baby is older and she is feeling more confident herself. However, during these first months, this fourth trimester (notice months, not weeks), she is the one who needs reassurance. So, to the partners, no matter how much you wish she would tear your clothes off and tell you how sexy you are, now is the time for you to tenderly reassure her that you find her attractive *as she is*. Be patient; your time will come.

Daniel, a father of one in Oklahoma, expresses the revelation that eased his worries, "At some point, it occurred to me that sex was not her first priority. That may sound like a no-brainer, but it helped." He found he could calm his own anxieties about whether his girlfriend still found him attractive, by reminding himself of her priorities.

Note to Partners: Patience and Understanding are the New Hot! Getting annoyed at the baby is a *turn-off*. Being understanding of her attunement to the baby is a *turn-on*.

What if you manage to do all the things necessary to facilitate a sexual encounter (you are rested enough, have had a shower, the baby is asleep, the bed is not full of baby poo or vomit, you are not mad at each other about who got up in the middle of the night for burping, etc.), and then the baby wakes up and interrupts you? If you can be understanding about the interruption, you are more likely to get another shot at this the next time the opportunity arises. It might be in five minutes when the baby is calm, or it may be another day. As Jessica in Fort Wayne, Indiana, told me at a conference: "When Allison understood my

connection to our baby, it made me feel more connected to her, too."
On the other hand, if you groan and complain, you are less likely to get
that second shot.

Figuring Out *When* and *Where* Are More Complicated than You Think Some babies sleep for long stretches of time, allowing the possibility of regular sexual encounters taking place in your own bed. Unfortunately, many babies do not sleep this much, and couples must engage their creative problem-solving skills when they want to have sex. One of the problems can be that most babysitters work in your home, especially if you have older children as well. Flex your resourcefulness and look for a relative, friend, or babysitter who will take care of your baby and older children at their house.

Another option, if you can afford it, is a hotel or, if you have access, a hot tub garden. Sometimes the chaos of your own home is a turn-off in itself. Think of a hotel room for an afternoon as the same price as dinner and a movie. It may be something you never did before having a baby, but you may find it to be a lovely in-town, get-away experience that you want to continue even when your children are older. Once a month, a babysitter, hotel, or other creative option like this, may well be well worth it for you and your partner.

Sex Can Hurt More after Having a Baby For more than half of all women, sex after giving birth is more painful than it was previously. You are far from alone if this describes you. The most common reason is vaginal dryness, so, generally, the first thing to try is more lubrication. The hormones that support lactation and suppress ovulation also tend to make our vaginas drier, even if we are aroused. If lubrication does not ease discomfort, some women find an estrogen cream helpful. This is a topical cream, not an estrogen pill taken internally, so it does not have the same effects on your body hormones that pills do. It is considered safe to use while breastfeeding and can make a world of difference in just a few weeks.

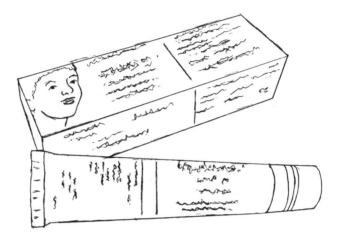

I have found, as have many other women, that natural lubrication improved the longer I breastfed my first child, and it was less of an issue following subsequent children. One theory is that your body is more efficient in hormone production and use as time goes on. If you plan to breastfeed long term, know that as your child starts to experiment with other foods besides breastmilk, you will probably see an increase in vaginal lubrication even though you are still lactating.

Often there can be more behind the pain than dryness. For some women, the way their stitches or tears heal can leave them with sensitive areas; for others, muscle spasms can occur that make sex painful. Solving these problems typically begins with an appointment with a care provider. Your care provider can evaluate how tears and stitches have healed, and either make recommendations for further steps to take, or help you find pelvic floor therapy. I know finding the time, energy, and money to make an appointment can be an obstacle, but I strongly urge you to consider it. Even if you do not intend to have sex for a while, you will feel better if you are actively making progress toward healing your perineum.

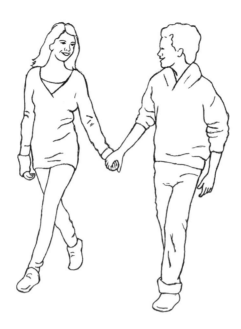

Feeling "Touched Out" is a Real Problem for New Mothers

Many new mothers who spend their days and nights caring for needy newborns want to spend their nonbaby time untouched. It's a serious mismatch for new mothers and their partners, who are likely feeling less touched than before the baby arrived.

There is no easy answer to this problem, although acknowledging the situation is a great start. Partners motivated to have more sex may find that providing down time without the baby encourages the new mother's receptiveness to touch. If you plan a date, you might also plan for the new mother to have several baby-free hours earlier in the day.

A new mother is likely to feel much more relaxed on a date if she's had time to shower and attend to herself without simultaneously caring for the baby. Partners may not realize how much time, effort, and care new mothers previously put into grooming and taking care of their bodies. As Angelika, from Dusseldorf, Germany, explains, "In the past, if I thought we were likely to have sex that evening, I would make sure to take a shower and get ready. You know, use lotions and perfume and put on make-up. If I can't do that earlier in the day, I just can't get in the mood later." And Cally, from Rutland, Vermont, wisely notes, "I didn't realize how much going to the gym helped my libido. It could be the exercise itself, but I think it was also just being in touch with my body. Like noticing that I even *have* a body. I can go weeks without noticing myself now."

Mothers and partners can become more conscious of making time for the new mother to be alone to take care of herself and her body. This is generally wonderful for new mothers, who can greatly benefit from a sense of autonomy, self-worth, and comfortableness with their changing bodies allowed by this time alone. It is also a valuable time for many women when they are looking to cultivate a mood for lovemaking.

Conclusion

Creating your new, postpartum sex life together requires patience and understanding. Ideally, within a relationship, we are able to express our real feelings, talk to each other openly, share our desires clearly, and make space for the ups and downs taking place in different areas of our relationship. All of us in partnerships know there is no "destination." We are always changing and seeking to change together.

Make sure you read chapters 3 (page 69) and 4 (page 105) discussing emotional health and the changing relationship with your partner. Maintaining a close emotional connection with your significant other, while taking care of yourself and your body, are key ingredients to enjoyable sex lives. When so much of your attention is focused on the cuteness you two have created together, it's easy to let your relationship, or your own health, take a backseat. Gently, slowly, you will become proficient at balancing all these things.

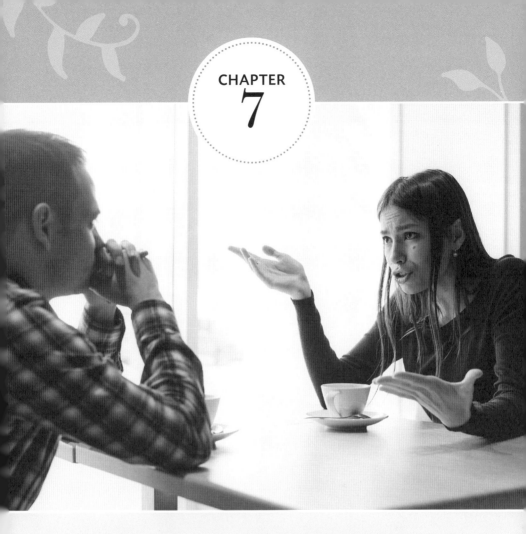

FOURTH TRIMESTER
EMOTIONS

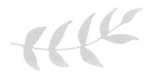

ALL WOMEN SHOULD SEEK TO BE ATTUNED to their emotional well-being in the postpartum period. Part of this new parenting period requires a constant "triaging" of needs. Too often, a new mother's own needs get shunted off behind the needs of others. In this chapter, there is a long list of ideas under the title "What Helps?" I encourage *all* new mothers to browse this list and implement suggestions that appeal to you.

To avoid depression and maintain our emotional well-being, we would all be wise to practice preventative healthcare. We can all benefit from choosing a few new healthy practices to incorporate into our lives, whether we are concerned about postpartum depression or not. Spending more time in nature, meeting other new parents, and exercising, regardless of our level of health, improve our lives in numerous ways.

When I set out to write this book, I searched online for information about the postpartum period. I was disappointed, but not surprised, to find that when I search for "postpartum" what turned up most frequently were the words "postpartum depression." On the one hand, "depression" is one of the most common terms we associate

> *We can all benefit from choosing a few new healthy practices to incorporate into our lives...*

with the word "postpartum." On the other hand, even though it is a phrase we easily piece together, most of us know very little about what postpartum depression is. Because there is not much understanding about the condition, most women with postpartum depression suffer in silence and isolation. It is even less well known that a traumatic birthing experience can result in PTSD, which is often mistaken for postpartum depression, even by some professionals. If you are concerned for yourself, your partner, or a friend, this chapter is designed to help you identify common symptoms and treatments that can offer relief.

Postpartum Emotional Well-Being

Major life transitions bring with them lots of emotions. Even though many of us are generally resilient or optimistic about change, we may experience a wider range of emotions at the time of life transitions. Births, deaths, marriages, divorces, graduations, and other milestones naturally encourage reflection on our lives. Sometimes sadness about a particular loss reappears during these events, even though it is not noticeable during more regular times.

Humans are complex emotional beings. Most of us harbor more levels of feelings than we normally acknowledge, unless we are in a therapist's office, deep in conversation with a good friend, or undergoing a major life transition. Then, nuanced layers of feelings may reveal themselves. I find it helpful to remind myself it is possible to be both happy and sad about the same event. For example, you may be ecstatic about the birth of your baby and simultaneously sad that your own mother could not be there. Maybe you feel closer than ever to your partner, who was an amazing support to you during labor, but also angry you ended up with a cesarean. All these emotions are real. One is not more genuine than the other.

Generally speaking, the presence of strong emotions—even emotions we consider negative, such as anger or sadness—is not a problem. Sometimes, our own judgment about what we "should" feel gets in the way of acknowledging how we do, truly, feel. That suppression, researchers say, can have a negative effect on us, including on our physical health.

I encourage you to embrace all the emotions of being a new parent. There are very few "shoulds" about how you feel in this raw and vulnerable time. Many women, even during pregnancy, find they weep easily at tear-jerking advertisements or stories. At the same time, we often experience renewed wonder at the world, as we see it through the eyes of our babies. Attend to your emotional well-being by practicing gentleness and acceptance toward your fluctuating sensations.

Emotional Well-Being Supports

1. What Helps? A Village

As a first step, think about how to increase the amount of support you receive, specifically as a mother to an infant. For some women, the issue is they are alone in a new city, or without relatives or friends. For others, the issue is they have trouble asking for or accepting help. Most women need help with baby care, especially with babies who cry a lot and do

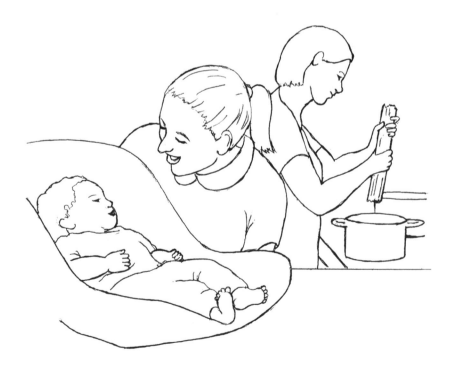

not sleep for long stretches of time. Even resilient mothers who once flourished while mothering other babies can find themselves stretched to their breaking point with a colicky, wakeful baby. New mothers feeling exhausted and overwhelmed may need more help with their household or business chores, which unfortunately do not go away just because you have a baby. Finally, some mothers may just need adult companionship and reassurance. While our pre-verbal babies are wonderful in their own way, they are not intellectually stimulating or able to offer genuine friendship. Women who are isolated and without a robust support system are at higher risk for postpartum depression.

Go to a Mother's Group If you're anxious or unmotivated to go to a group, ask a friend or relative to join you at a mother's group for your first time. I have co-led mother–baby groups in Ann Arbor for many years. One mother, who had just moved to Michigan during her third trimester, was suffering by herself and could not find the energy to research groups in the area. Her friend, who lived in California, found our group online and set up her friend's first visit to the group. Another mother, feeling traumatized by her birth experience, found some relief joining a mother–baby group and connecting with other mothers.

Rural Areas Rural women may have a harder time finding groups, but are no less in need of adult companionship. If this is you, see the table on pages 180–181 because many of these groups have local meetings in unusual areas. But you may have to get even more creative.

This is an area in which a partner, friend, or family member might be able to help by brainstorming about what is available and helping you utilize what you have. Are there churches, libraries, farmers' markets, co-ops, playgrounds, or other organizations in your area? They might not be "baby-centric," but they may allow you to find a few friends. One mother in rural Nebraska shared that she survived postpartum depression by forcing herself to visit her local library twice a week. It was a forty-five-minute drive, but she knew the librarian would warmly ask how she was and genuinely care to hear her answer. Another mother in Virginia drove half an hour to an indoor pool for parent–tot swim

Potential Support Groups in Rural Areas

Groups to Look For	What You'll Find	Where to Find Them
1. Local mother–baby groups	Usually led by an experienced doula, midwife, or social worker. Mothers take turns sharing, and strong bonds can form among group members.	Ask your pediatrician, midwife, or doula. Call the triage department at your hospital because it will often give out information about these local groups.
2. Mother–baby yoga class	Not just for the super-fit mothers who have been doing yoga for years before giving birth. As Jessica in Cleveland says, "There is usually a lot more socializing than doing serious yoga at those classes." It's a place to meet other mothers with small babies and soak up wisdom and calming mantras from the yoga instructor.	Ask at any local yoga studio. If they don't offer such a class, they will likely know who in your area does.
3. La Leche League	An international group, with local chapters, that focuses on breastfeeding support. Bottle-feeding mothers can often get great support here, too. Leaders are usually compassionate, informed, experienced mothers who want to support other mothers through the early weeks and months of a baby's life.	Visit the international website, www.llli.org, or ask your pediatrician, midwife, or doula.

Groups to Look For	What You'll Find	Where to Find Them
4. Hike-It-Baby	Hike-it-Baby groups meet all over the United States, Canada, and other places in the world. This group focuses on outdoor activities for parents with babies or small children.	Go to hikeitbaby.com.
5. Baby-wearing International	These groups meet with a certified leader knowledgeable about a variety of baby carriers (slings, wraps, etc.).	Go to babywearing-international.org.
6. MOMS Club	This group has local chapters and focuses on stay-at-home mothers. Meetings are held during the day and mothers can bring their children with them.	Go to momsclub.org.
7. MOPS	A Christian-centered group with regularly scheduled meetings. Mothers who join are assigned a mentor, and children are cared for during the meetings.	Go to mops.org.
8. Dancing for Birth	Although the name may sound like this group is only "for birth," this organization also includes postpartum mothers in its classes.	Go to dancingforbirth.com.

classes. When I asked online support groups for specific suggestions for rural dwellers, the most common suggestions were libraries and playgrounds.

For women struggling with postpartum depression, Catherine Fisher points out that if no group in your area fits you well, joining an online or text-based postpartum depression support group can be helpful. A 2015 study in St. Louis found that text messaging was a successful support option for mothers with postpartum depression. Specific support groups for postpartum depression exist on Facebook. Within these, be assured that the people reading your messages are empathetic to what you are going through.

Reach Out to Your Actual Neighbors In many areas, even if you haven't met them, your neighbors have likely noticed you were pregnant. Consider dropping off or mailing birth announcements to them. Some areas have the practice of putting up a temporary sign in the front yard, perhaps with balloons, that announces, "It's a Boy" or "It's a Girl." This can be a conversation starter that allows you to meet more neighbors or deepen a connection with those you've already met.

There may be neighbors who love babies or who remember their own postpartum days. Maybe a few will reach out to you. Even one good connection can be helpful.

2. What Helps? Exercise

In the first two weeks, you probably shouldn't do much more than go for a short walk for exercise. But as you recover from labor and delivery, longer walks are an excellent way to take care of yourself. In addition to the aerobic exercise, you also benefit from the sunshine. Exposure to sunlight ten to fifteen minutes a day is a proven mood booster. The chart on pages 180–181 includes several suggestions for group exercise ideas, such as yoga and dance. When I gave birth to my first child in New York City, I found that going swimming twice a week—and then soaking in a hot tub—did more for my mental health than just about anything else. I swam for thirty minutes, soaked for twenty, and the whole outing took about seventy-five minutes.

Bethany Drohmann, of Eugene, Oregon, was used to being very active before having her first child. After becoming a mother, she realized it was much harder to squeeze in physical activity. So she created "Mama Movement Cards" to help remind herself and other women to incorporate exercise into their daily lives. She suggests making movement simple, do-able, and part of an existing routine (such as when you are brushing your teeth or folding laundry). I have been inspired by her approach.

3. What Helps? Talk Therapy and Life Coaches

You do not have to be depressed or receive a clinical diagnosis to benefit from talk therapy or the support of a life coach. Life coaches help you identify goals, perhaps something as simple as, "I'd like to enjoy my time at home more and worry less about going back to work," and then find ways to make them happen. They help make you accountable for following through on what you want to do. Life coaches are sometimes less expensive than psychotherapists; however, they generally do not accept insurance as payment.

The two most common forms of talk therapy with psychotherapists or counselors are cognitive behavioral therapy (CBT) and interpersonal psychotherapy (IPT). These are the most common because researchers have studied them intensely and they are proven to work for many people. That said, other forms of therapy that might be less studied by researchers may work better for you.

Most people start with CBT or IPT because it is often covered by insurance. However, some people find great relief through art or music therapy, humanistic therapies such as Gestalt therapy, or integrative therapy that draws from a variety of approaches. These may not always be (but are sometimes) covered by insurance.

Make it a point to find a therapist with whom you can easily connect. This therapist is going to be a role model for how to speak to yourself, so make sure you feel good about the way the therapist speaks with you. If you do not have a positive first impression, continue searching. You deserve an empathetic connection.

Mama Moves by Bethany Drohmann

How we move all day, not just during an hour of exercise, is very important for health and well-being. Especially since having children, I find it of utmost importance to include small self-care movements with other routines. If I need to get my movement from an hour of dedicated exercise each day, but then forget about my body for the other twenty-three hours per day, I could be doing myself a huge disservice. I love having an hour (or more) of dedicated movement time alone and interrupted. I don't get too much of that these days, but relish it when I do, and try to ask for it when I desperately need it.

What keeps me sane, and what inspired me to make my deck of "Mama Moves Cards," is the fact that when we make something simple, do-able, and we associate it with specific routines, it is easier to do. If I stand on one leg to get some balance exercise while brushing my teeth, it is likely I will get my balance exercise done each day. If I remember to do some necks stretches while nursing, I will be better reminded to maintain healthy shoulder posture throughout the day. When I stand and type this, I am doing a calf stretch, which helps me remember my body and also get work done while I stretch.

Today, I have a six-week-old baby. I hold her a ton and nurse her throughout the day. One of the things keeping my body happier at the moment is that I have made it a habit to do one or two stretches immediately after I hand her to someone else. Another habit I have, which helps a lot, is folding laundry at a location that allows me to alternate a few hip stretches as I fold.

The Mama Moves I'm describing don't require extra time. I stay flexible, aware, and more relaxed throughout the day when I intersperse movement, alignment, and awareness among my daily tasks. And, because we remember things by association, I don't need to use extra brainpower to do any of it.

Find Bethany's "Mama Moves" cards at Mamamovescards.com.

Interpersonal psychotherapy is goal-oriented, short-term therapy rooted in the "attachment theory." That theory posits our original attachment to parents and care providers as an important key to our own self-image. This therapy, along with CBT, is taught widely in psychology and psychiatry programs. With the help of a practitioner, expect to explore how your relationships affect your mood, and vice versa, and to make steady progress toward goals you set at the beginning of therapy.

Cognitive behavioral therapy rests firmly on the concept that our feelings of fear or sadness arise because of the thoughts we have. For example, if I think to myself, "My boss is mad at me because I missed the project deadline and now I'm going to be in trouble," then I will likely walk into the next meeting with my boss feeling scared and anxious. CBT can help you identify the thoughts that come before your feelings, and give you tools to change those inaccurate or unhelpful thoughts. Using CBT, I might realize my feelings of fear in the preceding situation are not entirely warranted. Then, I might change my self-talk to something gentler: "My boss knows our team was asked to finish an additional project last week. I'm sure she will understand it is difficult to meet our deadline, and will react reasonably when I suggest we discuss a more realistic timeframe for the project." If I tell myself this instead of, "My boss is mad at me," I am likely to feel calmer about the situation.

Most of what we tell ourselves as new mothers is subconscious. Without even being aware of it, we may be telling ourselves things like, "All the other new moms look so happy. I'm a mess. There must be something wrong with me. I'm a terrible mother for wishing my baby weren't here so I could just get some sleep." Therapy helps us make those thoughts more conscious so we can ask ourselves whether there are more helpful, gentle things we could speak to ourselves instead. Therapy is a practice, I find, that helps most people treat themselves more like they treat other people—with kindness and compassion.

4. What Helps? Natural Mood Remedies

I prefer a natural approach to daily living. Whenever possible, I try to find natural remedies for my health needs before settling on more mainstream medicine. Scientific studies are paying more and more attention to natural remedies for our twenty-first century ailments. I believe the foods and herbs our ancestors used for healing their bodies are probably as effective, or sometimes more effective, than what we use now, even if scientists are just beginning to understand why.

Herbal Medicines If you are interested in learning more about herbs and how they may help you, speak with a trained herbalist who can help you understand the way a specific herb might affect you, and your baby through your breastmilk. Herbs are potent substances, and being in the care of an herbalist is wise if you are going to use them. The two most common herbs used for depression are St. John's Wort and SAMe (S-Adenosyl-L-Methionine). SAMe is an herbal supplement widely used in Europe and can be found over the counter in the United States. Neither of these herbs has been widely studied for their effects on babies through breastmilk; however, they are generally considered safe for use by breastfeeding mothers. Different herbs can interact in significant ways with pharmaceutical medication, so let your doctor know if you are thinking about using them.

Sunlight Exposure or Bright Light Therapy Studies show that bright light therapy helps people with seasonal affective disorder feel better. Pregnant women with depression have also shown improvement using this method. There is less data about postpartum use, but it is clear that *some* women feel better, while some women do not. If you are among those for whom it works, this could be a great solution.

Spend Time in Nature Being surrounded by trees or being able to gaze at a lake or ocean helps us instantly relax. This probably makes intuitive sense to you. I know that I feel better when I spend time outdoors in a natural setting. However, the research is compelling. University

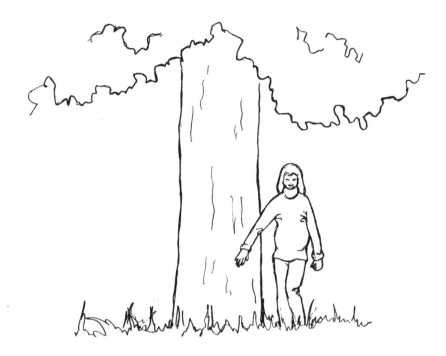

of Michigan researchers found that a single walk in a forest improved memory by 20 percent, compared to people who walked down a city street. Immune systems appear stronger after time in nature, even to the level of producing anti-cancer proteins. There are strong associations between longer lives and living near nature. The effect of nature on mood is magnified, apparently, if you spend time near natural water, like a lake or river. Go outside!

Nutritional or Vitamin Supplements (Especially Magnesium, Omega-3s, and Vitamin B$_2$) When you feel down, and have a new round-the-clock job (taking care of a baby), you may not be eating well. Our bodies create hormones and neural connections from the food we eat and the liquid we drink. So an ice cream binge is not going to help you as much as a serving of leafy, green vegetables or chia seed pudding. This might be an effective time in your life to consider supplements. Some studies show that therapeutic doses of omega-3s, especially from fish oil, have a beneficial impact on mothers suffering from depression. Taking other vitamins that include B_2 (riboflavin) also appears to be beneficial. What I've found most encouraging is that magnesium is being prescribed more often for breastfeeding mothers before other drugs. Our knowledge of dietary supplements is growing, and some fads seem to rise and fall rapidly, so it is worth consulting with experts in this area.

Acupuncture   Promising research about acupuncture's use during pregnancy makes it a safe treatment to try postpartum. Although some people are scared of the idea of needles, it helps to know that the needles are as thin and bendable as a strand of your hair. I recommend you find an office that uses sterile, one-time-use needles, which is the standard. Rather than feeling pain from the needles, many people who have experienced acupuncture describe a sensation of "floating" or "calmness." As someone who looks away with a grimace whenever I have to give blood, I can testify that acupuncture is entirely different. However, you may not find relief; some people do not. On the other hand, you may discover you are like thousands of others who do. Like all modalities, find a practitioner you like and trust.

Postpartum Depression

Postpartum depression (PPD) is different from mood swings described in chapter 1 (see page 13). Every new mother experiences the rise and fall of hormone levels as her body adjusts from pregnancy to lactation. This shift is made all the harder by lack of sleep caused by most labors and the wakefulness of most newborns. If you feel weepy and upset in the first two weeks postpartum, you are not alone. This is why most clinicians won't diagnose postpartum depression early on. In most cases, mothers can safely wait out those first two weeks to determine whether their moods begin to lighten. Birth and postpartum doula, Catherine Fisher, finds it helpful to share with her clients that PPD often makes it difficult to function—more so than the feelings, fears, and sleep deprivation that are normal to all new mothers. Postpartum depression will usually, but not always, surface later—in the weeks, and even months, following birth.

Alyssa, a new mother who attended our mother–baby group, said she had been warned about the hormone overload of the first week. After her milk came in, she kept waiting for her feelings of sadness and being overwhelmed to subside, but they never did. Finally, at five weeks postpartum, she reached out for help. If your feelings do not seem more manageable after two weeks or so, that is a good time to seek help. Luckily, postpartum depression has become increasingly well studied and understood. More and more practitioners specialize in treating it.

Suicide Hotline

If you or someone you know is in crisis, call 911 or the toll-free twenty-four-hour hotline of the National Suicide Prevention Lifeline at:

1-800-273-TALK (1-800-273-8255)
TTY: 1-800-799-4TTY (4889)

One caveat with this advice: If you have a history of depression or if your feelings are worrisome to you or your loved ones, *you should not wait* even two weeks. Especially if you recognize worrisome symptoms in yourself that you have experienced before, it's a good idea to contact your mental healthcare provider early. Most urgently, if your symptoms include suicidal thoughts, thoughts about harming yourself or your baby, an inability to eat, or hallucinations, seek help from a therapist or practitioner without waiting to see if these things get better on their own.

It's important to know that partners can experience postpartum depression as well. While PPD is under-diagnosed in biological mothers, it is even more misunderstood and under-diagnosed in new parents who did not give birth themselves. The stresses of adjusting to life with a newborn, and the changes to one's own life and self-image, affect the entire family. While partners used to be diagnosed with "clinical depression," the idea that there is a category of depression unique to the postpartum period related to living with an infant has been expanded to now include partners.

What to Look For

According to the National Institutes of Health, common PPD symptoms to watch for include the following:

- Feeling sad, hopeless, empty, or overwhelmed
- Crying more often than usual, or for no apparent reason
- Worrying or feeling overly anxious
- Feeling moody, irritable, or restless
- Oversleeping, or being unable to sleep even when your baby is asleep
- Trouble concentrating, remembering details, and making decisions
- Experiencing anger or rage
- Losing interest in once-enjoyable activities
- Suffering from physical aches and pains, including frequent headaches, stomach problems, and muscle pain
- Eating too little, or too much
- Withdrawing from or avoiding friends and family
- Having trouble bonding, or forming an emotional attachment with the baby
- Persistently doubting your ability to care for your baby
- Thinking about harming yourself or your baby

You do not need to experience all, or even most, of these symptoms to be affected by PPD. If you are experiencing strong feelings of sadness or hopelessness, for example, that alone can be the basis for seeking help.

Postpartum Depression: What Helps?

Usually, a combination of adjustments can help with PPD. These include all the ideas discussed previously: regular exercise, a strong support system, talk therapy or a life coach, mindfulness meditation, spending time in nature (especially in the sun), nutritional supplements, and herbs. In addition, medication exists specifically for postpartum depression. Some women may only need one of these solutions, while others will benefit greatly from combining three or four. The important thing is to find what works best for you, rather than struggling through each day by yourself. It is not good for you, nor is it healthy for your baby, for you to tough it out.

Medication

You may know from earlier life experiences that pharmaceutical medication helps you feel better, or this may be the first time you have considered using it. In either case, I strongly suggest incorporating some of these natural remedies into your routine. For some women, they are enough to relieve worrisome symptoms. For others, they support the work of medications.

There is definitely a time and place for pharmaceutical medication. For some who find relief using medicine for their depression, consistent long-term use is most beneficial. For others, short-term use may be appropriate. A compassionate therapist in my town views pharmaceutical use for postpartum depression as a tool to help a woman "get out from under." When she's feeling better, she may be able to use other coping mechanisms more fully.

Although not every talk therapist can prescribe medications, they should be able to refer you to a psychiatrist or psychiatric nurse who can. Talk to your provider about the possible effects of passing antidepressants or other medications to your baby through your breast-milk. While the major pharmaceutical drugs commonly prescribed for postpartum depression (tricyclic antidepressants, selective serotonin reuptake inhibitors, and estrogen) are passed to the baby through breastmilk, some are less worrisome than others. Estrogen, in particular, can have a negative effect on milk production. Remember that untreated depression also has an effect on your baby—so when weighing the effects of these drugs in your breastmilk, take that into account as well.

PTSD from a Birthing Experience

Some mothers experience something more than depression. Even less diagnosed and less treated than depression, post-traumatic stress from traumatic birth experiences is real, and often debilitating, for thousands of women. Robyn Brickel, a therapist in Alexandria, Virginia, explains that trauma can occur from these experiences:

- Any that overwhelms one's ability to stay grounded in the present, be mindful of one's environment, and/or tolerant of one's feelings
- Any in which the individual encounters (subjectively) a threat to life, body, sanity, or survival
- Any that includes a response of intense fear, helplessness, anger/rage, grief/betrayal

These criteria are too often present at childbirth. Estimates of PTSD prevalence range from 3 percent to 17 percent of birthing women.

One difference between postpartum depression and post-traumatic stress disorder is that mothers with PTSD often suffer from intrusive memories and flashbacks related to the traumatic event. They may find certain situations so triggering that they go out of their way to avoid them. It is also possible, and common, to experience depression and PTSD at the same time.

Most birth stories inspire me; however, I have heard about (and attended) a handful of births that have horrified me. Sometimes, it's the physical events that are scary, as in the case of a baby being whisked away to the NICU, a postpartum hemorrhage, or what is called a "stat" or "crash" cesarean. *The Atlantic* magazine ran a widely shared story in 2015 about birth-induced PTSD that featured the account of Sarah, a 28-year-old mother from Nebraska. Sarah unexpectedly gave birth seven weeks before her due date and her daughter was taken to the NICU before she could even hold her. By the time Sarah first saw her baby, there were "wires everywhere, a tube in her mouth," and when Sarah tried to touch her, "a nurse told her she was doing it wrong." A few months later she began to experience "anxiety, flashbacks, and other PTSD symptoms, even bursting out crying in her church group."

The Atlantic article was one step toward more awareness of this difficult and trying situation within our mainstream culture. However, it was unequipped to shed light on, what I have found to be, the largest category of women who experience birth-induced PTSD: women who are mistreated, demeaned, or dis-empowered by their care providers during pregnancy, labor, and/or delivery. How care providers speak with a woman, how they approach decision making (whether they believe intervention decisions are theirs to make alone, or whether they include the mother), and how a woman's body is touched or looked at all contribute to the birth experience—whether wonderful, or traumatic. The actions of a disrespectful doctor can lead to trauma; however, women who have experienced past trauma are more at risk of further trauma.

In the book, *Survivor Moms: Women's Stories of Birthing, Mothering, and Healing after Sexual Abuse* by Mickey Sperlich and Julia Seng, Sadie shares her experience of a vaginal exam during labor. She says, "During my son's birth, I had to handle a difficult invasion when the hospital doctor, who had been assigned to me, checked me for dilation. I knew that after he'd gotten the information he needed, he kept moving his finger inside me. It was repulsive. The nurses said later he often did that to women." (Page 101; used with permission.) Women in labor do not have the same ability to talk or fight back as they would normally, which contributes to feeling helpless and threatened.

The most famous case of abuse during childbirth in the United States occurred in 2013 to Kimberly Turbin. Video footage caught her physician cutting a brutal episiotomy against her will. The video has been viewed more than half a million times; news stories reached even more people as they flooded social media in 2015. She filed a lawsuit and eventually settled the case through legal mediation. Part of the reason Turbin settled and did not go to trial, according to Dawn Thompson, founder and president of ImprovingBirth, was that she was too upset about facing more years revisiting the traumatic event.

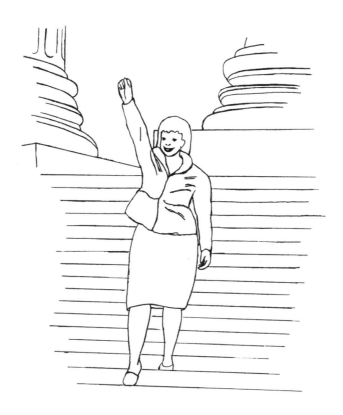

THE FOURTH TRIMESTER COMPANION

PTSD: What Helps?

Speaking Up Acknowledging our true feelings can be hard, even with ourselves. Sharing our true feelings with others can feel intimidating or scary. We can feel ashamed we are suffering with depression or post-traumatic stress. However, speaking up is powerful for the mental health of many women. There is the more public route of seeking legal remedy, which can help other women, too, as in Turbin's case. However, you can also lend your voice by writing a letter to your care provider, your hospital, or your provider's certifying board. This may be something you decide to do soon after your birth experience, or possibly much later. It is worth doing whenever you feel ready, even if it's years later! Writing in a journal is also proven to be effective in reducing worrisome symptoms.

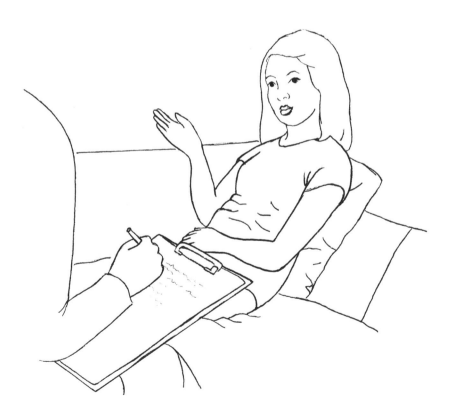

EMDR Women who experience PTSD can also benefit from the natural remedies and talk therapies listed previously for emotional well-being and aiding depression; however, they may not respond to the same medications. Another trauma-specific modality to try is EMDR (eye movement desensitization and reprocessing). This therapy involves moving your eyes from one side to the other while you briefly talk aloud about the triggering event. Researchers believe it works by allowing your unconscious mind to be involved in the "reprocessing" of the reminiscence, allowing it to recede into memory instead of remaining in a state of constant presence. Peggy Holtzman, M.S.W., is quoted in *Survivor Moms*, describing why she recommends EMDR.

> *I find EMDR to be a tremendous tool to help people heal from traumatic experiences . . . I have a perspective of the work both before and after being trained as an EMDR therapist. Before I was trained in EMDR, I found that healing would take place, but over a much longer period of time (i.e., months or years with a particular event vs. days or weeks using EMDR . . .). (Page 219; used by permission.)*

I know women who have found great relief through EMDR, so if you are suffering from PTSD symptoms, I believe it is well worth trying. In addition, for more daily maintenance, remember to add some gentle supports (such as time in nature, exercise, and herbal supplements) to your routine as well. I wish you much healing.

Conclusion

Having a baby is a major life transition and it is bound to stir up a lot of emotions. Some of us start off a bit fragile, because of our own childhoods or life experiences, and the experience of childbirth and becoming a parent may feel even more overwhelming or difficult than it does to others. Finding what works for us in this time will be a lifelong help. There will surely be emotional storms ahead, so if you learn that time in nature or writing in a journal or talking to a therapist helps you feel more steady and resilient now, you will be able to turn to these aids again. Remember that feeling sad, scared, or angry is part of being human, and these emotions can coexist alongside joy and happiness. Emotional well-being is not the absence of feelings, but the ability to live well with all your emotions. I hope you find some useful tips in this chapter for improving or enhancing your ability to find joy and peace.

THE FOURTH TRIMESTER COMPANION

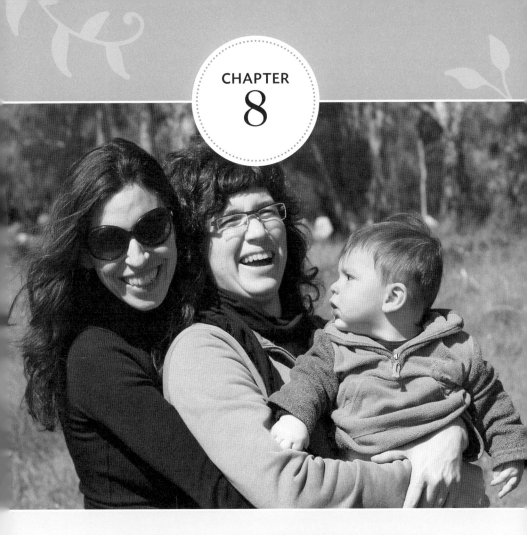

EMERGING FROM THE FOURTH TRIMESTER COCOON

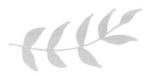

B Y NECESSITY, MOST OF YOUR ATTENTION DURING this fourth trimester is directed at nurturing yourself, your baby, and, if you have a partner, your primary relationship. However, other concerns beyond the "nest" often intrude into our sacred space. As early as the end of pregnancy, some women find themselves confronted by a friend's or co-worker's judgment of the decision to stay home, or return to paid employment, after having a baby.

Other mothers know they will have to travel with (or without) their infant soon after giving birth. And, though fertility concerns may seem far away to pregnant women, questions about a return to fertility usually pop up in the first weeks after giving birth.

This chapter is designed to help women for whom these issues arise during the fourth trimester and aid others as they look ahead. Hold your baby on your lap, sip from a glass of water, and browse any section that might be of use to YOU. I wish you a peaceful and smooth transition from the fourth trimester into the rest of your life as a parent.

> *...a division between stay-at-home mothers and mothers in the paid workforce is a detrimental division to us all.*

Fertility and a Return to Menstrual Cycles

Another concern new mothers face is managing their fertility in the postpartum period. Some women need to confront the question of birth control as early as four or five weeks postpartum; others do not regain fertility for more than a year. Wherever you are on this spectrum, you will, no doubt, be thinking about it during your fourth trimester.

A Quick History of Spacing Children

As an anthropologist, I find it fascinating that evidence suggests our ancestors were able to space their children about four years apart for millions of years without any artificial contraception. In college classes, when I ask undergraduates to hypothesize how they were able to do this, it usually takes fifteen or more guesses before someone hits upon the answer. They posit whether our ancestors had infrequent sex, whether they employed the "pull-it-out" method, or whether their diets were inadequate for getting pregnant. All are good guesses; however, anthropologists believe that breastfeeding was the real answer.

For most of human history, we were foragers (otherwise called gatherer–hunters) and walked long distances as part of normal life. It's very likely most children were not able to take part in the necessary walking on their own until they were about four years old. Spacing children about four years apart helped everyone survive better because adults had fewer children to carry at one time. Over a lifetime of fertility, this spacing meant that women might have about four to six children. It also meant that women had relatively few periods during their lifespan.

Exclusive breastfeeding suppresses the hormones that stimulate ovulation. For this suppression to occur, milk needs to be removed from the breast many times a day without any large time breaks between sessions. Five hours between feedings is approximately the longest break that can occur during the day while still maintaining this suppression. Some sources say suppression can be maintained if there is no milk removal for six hours at night. When you experience breaks longer than five or six hours, your body receives the message that your baby is less dependent on your breastmilk and, therefore, it is okay to get pregnant again.

Foraging, as a lifestyle, is much more compatible with exclusive breastfeeding than is agriculture. Foraging women usually had their babies and toddlers close by and only "worked" a few hours per day. When humans developed farming about 10,000 years ago, they had to work in conditions far different than those of foragers. During planting and harvesting seasons, lactating women had to work long hours. They might be away from their children for many hours each day, for several days in a row. As a result, farm families had far more children, sometimes spaced as close together as nine or ten months.

Using Lessons from Foragers to Delay Ovulation

If you hope to delay ovulation, think more like a forager than a farmer. Aim to breastfeed frequently, without long breaks between sessions. The medical term for this phenomenon of suppressed ovulation as birth control is "lactational amenorrhea method" or LAM. Ovulation is the release of an egg from a woman's ovary, and it occurs approximately two weeks before the period in a menstrual cycle.

Miriam Labbok, of Gillings School of Global Public Health at the University of North Carolina, Chapel Hill, examined evidence about the contraceptive use of breastfeeding. In the December 2015 issue of *Clinical Obstetrics and Gynecology* (vol. 58, no. 4, pp. 915–927), she wrote that women who breastfeed exclusively and frequently for six months have a greater than 98 percent chance of avoiding pregnancy, which is the same rate that most oral contraceptives achieve in practice.

After the first six months, many families start to supplement breastmilk with other food. To maintain LAM, no more than 10 percent of a baby's diet can come from other food. Clearly, for our ancestors, breastmilk made up the bulk of children's diets for a long time. Breastfeeding also has to maintain its frequency and intensity. Some babies cooperate with this and eagerly breastfeed for a year or two; other babies sleep longer or develop an increased interest in table food. Studies find that pumping milk does not regulate hormones in the mother's body quite the same way as breastfeeding. In some mothers who pump, cycles may return sooner than they would otherwise. In the modern era, women have to be aware of the signs that show cycles are returning once they begin to pump or after introducing table foods.

If you do not breastfeed exclusively, you can return to fertile status quickly. About 50 percent of women who do not breastfeed their babies exclusively will ovulate before six weeks have passed.

Recognizing Fertility Signs

Some women are familiar with fertility signs because they tracked their cycles to become pregnant. Many other women, especially women on long-term hormonal birth control, have never paid close attention to fertility signs before. Generally speaking, there is one easy way to recognize that your body is returning to its normal cycles and that you will be able to get pregnant again: the presence of fertile mucous. This is the sign to look for—not the return of menstruation.

Right after having a baby, you experience vaginal bleeding for several weeks. When this passes, if you pay close attention, you should notice very few vaginal secretions. In the previous section discussing postpartum sex (see page 171), I noted that vaginal dryness is an issue for many women. Dryness occurs as a side effect of the hormones that support lactation and suppress ovulation.

When you ovulate, there is a dramatic shift in vaginal secretion. Your cervix creates mucous usually described as "like an egg white." If you touch it with your fingers, it is sticky and extremely stretchy—like an egg white. This is "fertile mucous." Its design and structure assist semen, if it is nearby, to move upward. In other words, this fertile mucous not only signals you have ovulated, it actively helps you get pregnant if semen is introduced into your vagina.

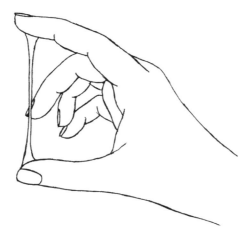

Important!

So, you *are able* to get pregnant even if you have *not yet had a period.* This is important for all women to understand. Relying on your first period to tell you that you are able to get pregnant is too late. Fertile mucous is a more reliable indicator.

If this method creates concern or anxiety, use a back-up contraceptive method. However, you should know that noticing fertile mucous postpartum is often easier than during regular cycles. During your regular cycle, vaginal secretions appear throughout the entire cycle. But postpartum, the change is normally quite dramatic—from virtually no secretions at all (during suppression) to fertile mucous (when you have ovulated).

If you want to rely on natural birth control methods, learn more about them at a variety of online websites. If you plan to have more children, sometimes the time between babies is a chance to experiment with natural birth control with more ease than at times when you are sure you are not ready for another baby. Marcie, a mother of one in Brooklyn, New York, had been on the pill since high school, before she decided to have children. She told me when she resumed her cycle fourteen months after having her son, it was the first time in her life she was able to track her cycles and notice fertility signs. Even though her cycle was unpredictable for a full year, she always knew when she was ovulating because she noticed fertile mucous. She said, "Because I wanted another child at some point, I wanted to stay off the pill. If I got pregnant, I wouldn't mind, but actually, it worked better than I imagined and I didn't get pregnant until we tried *during* the time of fertile mucous. Then I got pregnant immediately." Marcie is certain she only wants two children, and feels confident that a combination of fertility awareness and condoms (during her fertile times) will be her future birth control method.

If you decide to use a fertility awareness method as your birth control, be aware that women often track their daily temperature, in addition to fertile mucous. Some methods also recommend tracking cervix position. These fertility awareness methods are very effective when used correctly. Keep in mind, however, that women with newborns often find themselves waking at different times each morning, which can throw off daily temperature readings.

New technology promises to make reading our bodies' signs easier and faster. A fertility monitor called OvaCue uses saliva to predict and then confirm that ovulation has occurred. If you are interested in learning more about natural fertility mothods, I recommend the classic book, *Taking Charge of Your Fertility,* by Toni Weschler.

Postpartum Birth Control

Most care providers will talk to you about your plans for birth control during your six-week checkup. As I've already noted, if you are not breastfeeding exclusively, you may need to think about birth control even before that visit. Although it's hard to find exact numbers, research suggests that most women change their birth control strategies after

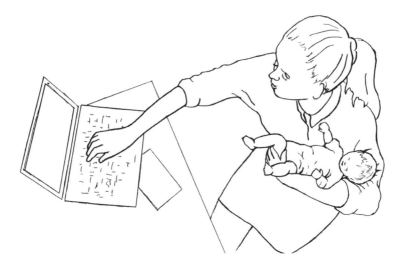

having children. What fit into your life before, may not fit well now. Take time to research this *before* your six-week visit, so you can pose any questions you need answered. A good resource for information about a wide variety of birth control options is the book and the website *Our Bodies, Ourselves* (ourbodiesourselves.org). Be open to trying something different that might fit with your life as a new mother.

Mommy Wars

An issue you may begin to face in the fourth trimester, that often extends far beyond, is the division between stay-at-home mothers and mothers who return to paid employment. Our culture does not honor or value parenting very highly, and I believe that is an underlying factor in these "Mommy Wars."

In the United States, like nowhere else in the world, this divide among women exists and hurts us all. The truth is, we are trapped in an all-or-nothing system. Many of us have to decide between not getting paid at all, or returning to full-time paid employment within a few days or weeks of giving birth to retain benefits and seniority. Although part-time employment might seem like the ideal choice between these options, because of the structure of U.S. healthcare, so often tied to full-time employment, many women cannot realistically take advantage of part-time work.

This black-and-white choice is hard on many of us. The stories that many women shared with journalist Catherine Pearson for the *Huffington Post* article "Here's Why Family Leave is a Huge Deal for New Parents," are heartbreaking. Instead of criticizing the *choice itself*, some women spend their time judging another woman's decisions.

One solution to these so-called "Mommy Wars" is increased exposure to stories about a possible third option: extended family leave. It's likely many of us in the United States would choose extended family leave if it were available. Instead of arguing about which option between our current two is right or better, let's talk more about expanding our options.

In many other countries, governments do not see extended leave as a benefit for the parents, but as a benefit to the child, who is their new citizen. There are many ways a child can gain from extended leave, firstly by allowing parents to be less financially stressed while taking care of their newborn. One study shows that children perform better in school when their fathers took paternity leave during their first year of life. Another found decreased infant mortality in the first year of life when parents had more time at home in the first year.

U.S. Surgeon General, Regina Benjamin, saw extended leave as a public health benefit because it allows many more mothers to breastfeed beyond a few short weeks. Extended leave allows mothers to be relaxed about breastfeeding their six-week-old. That mother does not have to feel stressed about pumping every day, building up a freezer supply of milk, and getting her infant to take a bottle before she is gone for forty hours a week. She can work on her breastfeeding relationship with her infant, and not on making that relationship bend to the demands of her employer.

Certainly, children's health in our nation would be improved if more babies could be breastfed, and could be breastfed longer than they currently are. Surgeon General Benjamin wrote a "Call to Action" in 2011 that specifically promotes paid family leave as an important way to increase breastfeeding rates. So far, only California, New Jersey, and Rhode Island have state laws mandating parental leave.

I had long heard about the positive experiences with parental leave in Europe, Russia, and Canada from friends. For example, a friend in Sweden gave birth to her daughter and shared 480 days of leave with her husband. She writes, "I don't know how anyone does it without leave. I am sure we would have divorced without having that time together while we struggled to figure out what we were doing." As mentioned in an early chapter, the photographer Johan Bävman has created a powerful photography exhibit about Swedish fathers who participate in parental leave (www.johanbavman.se/swedish-dads/).

When I had my second child in Toronto, Canada, I experienced first-hand how a national paid family leave program affected women's relationships with each other—and, frankly, with themselves. In New York, while I attended mother–baby support groups with my first baby, I felt a strong division between the mothers going back to paid work soon, and those staying home. Friendships seemed to fall along these fault lines. The mothers going back to a job had to focus a lot of their time and

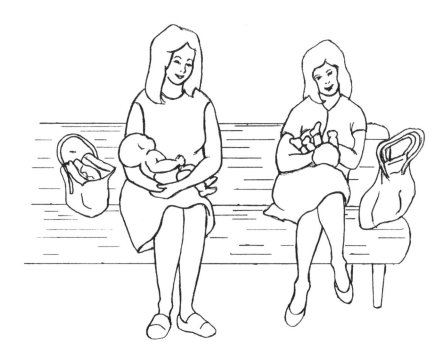

attention on pumping and bottle-feeding questions. The anxiety was palpable to everyone.

In Toronto, where I had my second child and our family enjoyed a year of paid leave, I was astonished and delighted when other parents I met at the park or at drop-in centers would talk about my new baby and also inquire about my profession. Even with tiny newborns in carriers, I found myself chatting with women about their careers and interests. The fact that I was simultaneously caring for a newborn and also sending out job applications was treated as normal. I found I loved this mixing of identities and, when I returned to the States, missed this almost most of all.

Paid leave in Canada allows mothers and fathers to be both stay-at-home parents and have a career. It is safe and normal to talk about both parts of your life. Nobody judges anyone else as having made the wrong choice for the child or for women's rights. Some parents do decide to extend their leave and stay at home longer than a year, but, if they do, they do not have to sacrifice their professional identity. It's part of the culture to assume parents are both parents and workers.

I know funding parental leave is a political hot potato, but I want to suggest, wherever you fall politically, you recognize that a division between stay-at-home mothers and mothers in the paid workforce is a detrimental division to us all.

Our culture requires most of us to choose more definitively between spending time with our newborn or continuing our career—and we must make this choice far earlier than we are comfortable. I think most of us are unwitting participants in the "Mommy Wars," afraid of being judged for our own choices and, therefore, silenced. The more we realize how differently this choice plays out in other countries with more extensive leave policies, the less we might be inclined to judge parents in our own country. Our choice is heavy, and more absolute, with little room for creativity or compromise because we don't have a "both/and" option.

The message that employers and governments send when there is no option for parental leave, or only unpaid leave, is that taking care of a baby is not important. This message must be challenged and revised.

At the end of one mother–baby group at the Elizabeth Seton Birth Center in New York City, Ellen Chuse once said, "I won't see you for a week, and it may seem like what you do in this next week is not important. You'll change diapers, feed your baby, and try to get enough sleep. But I want you to know that what you are doing is *very* important. It is the most important job in the world. If I could, I would rearrange the powers-that-be so *you* got paid like CEOs, because what you're doing is changing the world. Every day. You are making the world a better place by raising kind and thoughtful and loving people. You deserve a million bucks."

Although I don't know how to fund it, I concur with Ellen. I look forward to, and I am working toward, a world in which parenting is rightfully valued and acknowledged. If you have a career or important activities that are part of who you are, you will naturally bring that richness to your parenting, creating a unique parenting style fit for your family and your children. Whether traditional or progressive, you *are* making the world a better place by choosing to be a thoughtful, hardworking, and loving parent.

Traveling

Around October, the mothers in my mom–baby groups always begin sharing their anxieties about traveling with a baby during the holidays. I grew up as the oldest of seven children in a military family, so traveling long distances with babies was part of normal life for me. Even so, I got the jitters when I became a new mother and faced several trips in my daughter's first year of life. I feel blessed that our first big trip was by train, from New York to Washington, D.C., and I was able to hold her and give her my undivided attention the entire trip. This gentle start to traveling helped me gain confidence. Next, we went on a plane trip to Germany when she was three months old, and then to Russia when she was ten months old, and from New York to California when she was one year old. Hopefully, the fact that I survived all these trips will inspire you to try traveling with young ones.

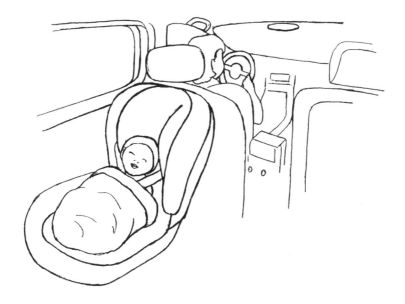

We all know how to prepare for our own successful trip, but how do we prepare to bring along a small creature who often cries, occasionally blows out a diaper, and potentially breastfeeds for hours at a time?

Let me start by saying I love traveling with infants under one year of age. Infants who cannot crawl are my favorite traveling companions. Given the choice, I would travel around the world three times over with a six-month-old before I would travel 20 miles (32 km) with a toddler. Toddlers are typically much more difficult to bring on trips than babies who cannot yet walk. Toddlers have an intrinsic need to move around, and do not yet have the required attention span to spend multiple hours watching videos. In addition, they are generally more attached to bed-time routines, and harder to put to sleep on an airplane or in a car. Babies, on the other hand, love to spend hours on your lap.

Long Car Trips

Most babies do not love car seats while you are driving around town. I know some mothers who honestly dread putting their baby in the car just to drop off older children at school or go to the grocery store. They are guaranteed a crying jag for those in-town trips. Yet many parents are pleasantly surprised by how much their babies are willing to sleep on long car rides. A surprising number of babies, including those who generally do not take long naps, will sleep for long stretches of time on highway drives. This is no guarantee, of course, but I would approach a car ride with the expectation you will have at least some hours of sleeping, and that those hours will be longer than being at home.

Long Car Trip Tips

- Plan on the trip taking significantly longer than Google Maps predicts!
- Break trips into shorter legs.
- Pump gas while your baby is awake so you can drive through long sleeping periods without stopping.
- Think about what time of day you will drive: Evening and night drives can be great!
- If you have two drivers, plan to spend part of the trip in the backseat, near the baby.

Plan on the Trip Taking Significantly Longer than Google Maps Predicts! You will, undoubtedly, need to make more stops when travelling with a baby. If adults tend to stop every three to four hours, you might expect to stop every two hours or so with a baby who is awake. (While she's asleep, drive, drive, drive!)

Break Trips into Shorter Legs We often choose to drive instead of fly to save money, especially now that we have three children. While spending the night at a hotel feels like an expensive luxury for a car trip that would take eight to twelve hours of driving, it can save your sanity to do so and will feel worth the extra expense. Pack your bathing suits! Most babies love water, and it can feel so relaxing to take your baby into the hotel pool after a day of driving.

If your car trip is less than eight hours, think of it as two chunks of time. Even longer trips can be broken up into smaller, manageable stretches. One of our common trips to the east coast from Michigan takes about twelve hours. That's two six-hour days (which is four three-hour trips). If we get an early start for the first chunk (driving 7:00 a.m. to 10:00 a.m.) we can have a long lunch and crawling-around baby playtime. Then, we get back in the car for the baby's late afternoon nap and drive from 1:00 p.m. to 4:00 p.m. We stop for dinner on the first day and, if things are going well, we might try to sneak in an hour or two of driving in the evening to make the second day easier. If you plan ahead for a fun daytime stop, like a library with a large children's section, or a kid's museum, you'll have a relaxing and rejuvenating break.

Pump Gas While Your Baby Is Awake So You Can Drive through Long Sleeping Periods without Stopping
If your baby wakes up because you stop for gas, you will only kick yourself.

Think About the Time of Day You Will Drive: Evening and Night Drives Can Be Great!
If your baby has a relatively early bedtime, you might be able to get a few painless hours on the road by leaving in the evening. It's up to you whether you put your baby to sleep at home, and then buckle him into the car seat, or whether you try to help him fall sleep on the road. You can decide what works best for your baby. Pack a dinner for the car and hit the road at 6:30 or 7:00 p.m. If your baby is asleep, you might even have some adult conversation without interruption.

Eltine DeYoung, a doula in Kalamazoo, Michigan, remembers, "When the kids were little, we always planned to drive most of the journey at night. Kids always slept for hours on end. When waking up we would stop for a quick bathroom break and we provided them with a homemade sandwich and other goodies while continuing on our way. During the day, many more stops were required as well as entertainment."

If you are driving to see grandparents or relatives eager to see your children, Jasmine, mother of two from the Upper Peninsula of Michigan, points out that if you drive at night, you can plan a nap the next day while your relatives care for your children. If you're awake and doing well in the evening, and near a populated area with many hotels, you can drive until 11:00 p.m. to get a good part of your driving done.

If You Have Two Drivers, Plan to Spend Part of the Trip in the Backseat, Next to the Baby If you expect to sit in the front seat the whole way, talking to your partner or listening to the radio, you will probably be disappointed. However, if you plan to spend a lot of the trip riding in the backseat with your baby, you will probably be able to help your baby stay happy and entertained. You will be more able to sing and talk to your baby, switch out toys, make faces, and otherwise keep her occupied while she is awake—and you will have an easier time feeding her.

Bring a cooler for bottles of milk. You can sometimes find free ice for your cooler at fast-food drive-throughs or gas stations. Bottles work easily in the car, of course. If your baby doesn't use a bottle yet, bring along a supplemental nursing system to finger-feed your baby (see page 97). Most babies who do not know how to suck from a bottle have success with the finger-feeding method.

Do not try to breastfeed your baby in the car seat by bending over her. Although this seems like a good idea, and it's even possible to do with the mother's seatbelt in place sometimes, a crash would send your body straight into your baby. That energy, at 30 miles (48 km) per hour—not even taking into account highway speeds—is deadly force.

Plane Trips *Without* Your Baby

Pumping in the Airport No matter how you try to arrange life and work, there are times when traveling without your infant is unavoidable. If you are back in the paid work force and still breastfeeding your baby, you are probably in the habit of pumping every few hours. How can you pump while you travel?

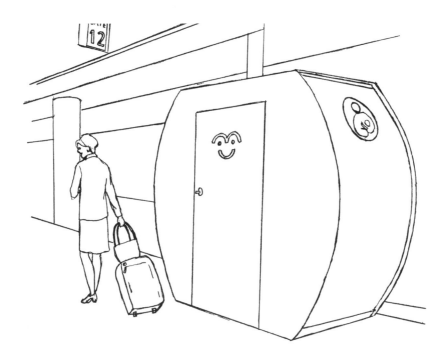

More and more international and American airports offer nursing and pumping stations. Some are rooms, such as the Mother's Room on Concourse C of Chicago O'Hare Airport, and some are moveable pods, such as the ones made by an innovative company called Mamava. These pods are located at a number of airports, but also in athletic stadiums, universities, and large businesses. You can find a list of participating U.S. airports on this website, including a map of where the stations are located: https://momaboard.com/traveltip/airport-nursing-rooms-united-states.

Pumping on the Plane Under normal circumstances, I am a strong advocate of a nursing mother's right to a clean, safe place to pump that is not in a bathroom. On a plane, though, many mothers decide to pump in the washroom. If this is your plan, think ahead and try to pump before drink service or meal service. Immediately after meals, the line for the bathroom is usually quite long.

I've also read many online descriptions of women pumping in their airplane seats. If that's something you feel comfortable doing, you will be in great company. However, I have two suggestions: Wear a hands-free pumping bra beneath your clothing so your breasts are already pump-accessible, and have a coat or blanket nearby to lay over you for added privacy. The loud noise of airplanes helps drown out the sound of your pump, but you might wait until most people around you are wearing earphones to watch a movie or listen to music.

Bring alcohol wipes with you to clean pump parts that come into contact with your milk. Do not rinse your equipment in the plane's bathroom sink. This water is often not safe to consume. On long flights, this might mean you have to dump a later pumping because you weren't able to clean some parts, but it will be safer for your baby.

If you do plan to pump onboard, your breast pump may be considered a "medical device." In this case, you are technically allowed to bring it along with two carry-ons. Your cooler will always be considered a carry-on. However, the TSA website does not specifically list breast pump as a medical device exception, and the Centers for Disease Control and Prevention website (cdc.gov) refers to breast pumps as a "personal item." For this reason, it is useful if your pump and cooler are in one bag, so they count as one carry-on.

Of course, the smaller and more portable your breast pump is, the better. I personally recommend the Medela Swing maxi double electric breast pump for pumping onboard a plane. When I taught at a university, I needed something small and lightweight with a strong pump. It fit in my purse easily and pumped as much milk as the larger, hospital-grade pump I kept at home.

Traveling with Pumped Milk When you travel, decide ahead of time whether you want to freeze milk from the entire trip and keep it frozen, or whether you will save just the milk you pump the last day of the trip. It's difficult to keep breastmilk frozen on a plane. Fresh breastmilk will keep in a cooler with ice for twenty-four hours—after that, it needs to be used or frozen. If you decide to freeze the milk you've pumped during a trip, book a hotel room with a freezer large enough for several bags of milk and frozen cooler bags. As you travel, it's likely you will need to refresh the ice frequently. Most airport restaurants and coffee shops are happy to help with this, as are flight attendants on long flights.

You may wonder whether you can carry breastmilk with your carry-on luggage, as there are strict guidelines for other liquids (no more than three fluid ounces, or 90 ml). Breastmilk is an exception to the liquids rule and you are allowed to carry more than three fluid ounces (90 ml). You can carry breastmilk whether you are traveling with or without your baby.

TSA agents may want to inspect your breastmilk and freezer packs. If so, you have the right to ask that they put on new, clean gloves to do so, and that they use fresh explosive-detection swabs. There is less strenuous screening for freezer bags and breastmilk that are frozen solid, rather than in a slushy or thawed liquid state.

Plane Travel with Your Baby

Congratulations! Your baby's flight likely did not cost you much if he is under two years of age. This is the best time to travel by plane! Still, you are probably concerned about how other passengers will respond if your baby cries, and you may also be worried about receiving disapproving looks or comments if you breastfeed. Do you remember that old advice to think of everyone in the audience wearing underwear when you're afraid to speak in public? Look around. I find it comforting to think about how many men and women on the flight have probably flown with a small child themselves. Take a deep breath.

Book Early to Request a Bulkhead Seat
Seasoned international traveler, Amy Allington, who worked in Moscow and traveled to the United States several times a year, swears by bulkhead seating. This area has more space and the added advantage that you are not kicking or pushing into the seat in front of you. Some large planes even have a baby bassinet that fastens to the bulkhead wall. If your baby is one to sleep in a bassinet, as Amy's babies did, this can be great. However, it can also be useful for holding all your baby gear within arm's reach while the baby is on your lap.

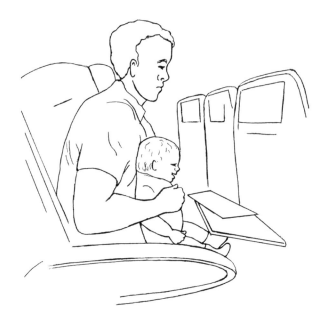

You Can Bring a Stroller All the Way to the Gate and Check It at the Gate Double-check with your airline, but most airlines do not count a stroller as extra baggage. I found it useful to bring a stroller, but actually wear my baby. The stroller carried our diaper bag, purse, and carry-on. That way my baby stayed calmer through the whole airport experience. There were even times TSA let me walk through the machines with my baby in the sling. Most of the time, this did not work, but when it did, it was wonderfully convenient!

Rent or Buy a Special Seatbelt for Your Baby Online and Be Aware Every Airline Has Its Own Rules About Take-Off and Landing There are special baby harnesses available, for rent or purchase, that attach to your own seatbelt. If you rent online, typically, the owner will send it to you before your trip, along with an envelope to send it back in afterward. If you have this device, I found many flight attendants will leave you alone during take-off and landing. Without it, however, I was given many more directions about what I must do with my child on my lap (including, "You can't breastfeed during take-off and landing."). Different airlines have different rules, sometimes completely contradictory. There's little you can do about this, but, hopefully, you will be less stressed if you know about it ahead of time.

Be Confident in Breastfeeding on Flights Take in the supportive words or glances, and ignore the haters. After all, you are feeding your baby! Just like most adults have a drink and snack or meal onboard a plane, your baby deserves to eat as well. Breastfeeding during take-off and landing (if allowed) might help while your baby's ears acclimate. Throughout the flight, it's probably your best calming tool. Even the haters are certain to prefer your baby happy and breastfeeding to screaming and crying. If you are comfortable warning your immediate neighbors at the beginning of the flight that you are a breastfeeding mother, they will have the chance to switch seats if they prefer. You can then be assured your seatmates are supportive—or, at the least, not offended.

Stay Hydrated! Bring a one-handed water bottle with a lid. It's hard to manipulate those wide-mouthed plastic airplane cups with a baby in arms, so you may be tempted not to drink anything at all. A better idea is to bring an empty water bottle with you and ask the flight attendant to pour your drink into it.

Accept Offers of Help This is no time to insist on doing all things yourself. If someone offers to carry your bag or lift it into the overhead compartment, please do yourself a favor and accept the help. Some wonderful people even offer to hold your baby. I think it is wise to have as many allies as possible on the flight, in case your baby ends up crying later. Psychologically, it can feel like you have supporters on board.

Bring Earplugs If your baby does cry on board, you might consider earplugs for yourself. I don't recommend this so you won't hear your own baby crying. I believe it helps you feel some distance from the people around you, in case you worry about judgment. Look for supporters! They are out there. There are other mothers or fathers on board who have flown with crying children before. Hopefully, they will make eye contact or otherwise show support. Remember how this feels, and for the rest of your life, make eye contact with parents of babies on flights and give them a thumbs-up. It's just good karma.

Conclusion

Your fourth trimester will end faster than you can imagine. Though at times each day might feel like a year, I know when you are launched into the fourth month and beyond you will likely look back on this time as a whirlwind.

Enjoy every moment you can in these early days and weeks with your newborn. Be gentle with yourself, your partner, and your extended family. Although parenting is a role that countless generations before us have fulfilled, we can feel alone and helpless when it is our turn. The cute moments are delightful, of course. When your baby smiles, laughs aloud, or makes a new discovery ("Hey! This is my hand! I am moving this hand! Look at me!"), parenting can easily feel like the best and easiest job in the world. But there are other moments, too, that challenge us, sometimes deeply. We may not have enough sleep to be patient or enough time to ourselves to feel normal. In the challenging times, it is easy to doubt yourself and worry that you are doing everything wrong.

I hope the stories here will help you will feel more able to appreciate the wondrous moments and also feel less alone during the challenging ones. You start to put your parenting philosophy into practice in the fourth trimester, but the relationship that is born out of this will last the rest of your lives. Good parent–child relationships are the fundamental building blocks of all societies. Though it may feel like insignificant work, as you fold baby clothes and soothe a crying baby at 3:00 a.m., I firmly believe you *are* making the world a better place by being a parent. Thank you for doing this important job.

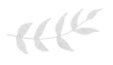

Acknowledgments

Helen McCabe
Crescent Moon Group
Felix Paulick
Phil Pianelli

Chelsea, Erin, Georgia,
Gracie, Meredith, Regan, Renee,
Shreya, and Tonia.

Garrett Potter
Cathy Reisfield
Meadow Snyder-O'Brien

Emily Adama
Mary Burke
Margo Lowenstein

Toni Aucker
Nicole Babbitt
Heather Boyd
Jennifer D'Jamoos
Bethany Drohmann
Jessica English
Anna Fernandez
Catherine Fischer
Martha Hollis
Lisa Klopfer
Jessica Lipiec
Ana Paula Markel
Gillian McClinsey-Powell
Melissa Palma
Garrett Potter
Barbara Robertson, IBCLC
Merilynne Rush
Mickey Sperlich
Tammy Twaddle
Kara Zahl

Amy Allington
Zoe Clarkwest
Tracey D'Arsie
Debi Fairman
Brenda Gabriel
Cheri Gabriel
Scott Gabriel
Lavetta Griffin
Theresa Smyth
Amy Tatko
Alex Vamos
Jennifer Woodill
Kary Young

Aiden Standke
Julie Wilson
Tabitha Wisecup

Anju

Sylvia

Calvin

Wendy Abate
Joseph Allen
Susie Allington
Cynthia Barry
Shannon Baer

Andrea Beals
Jean Bigelow
Diane Black
Celeste Craig
Cindy Harrington

Daryl Honor
Martha McDowell
Tara McKnight
Sarah Price
Perla Schaeberle

Jeff Schwartz
Amy Wallerstein
Margarete Walsh
Ruthie Wawtza
Ron Zang

About the Author

Cynthia Gabriel, Ph.D., is mother to three, a birth and postpartum doula, childbirth educator, and medical anthropologist. Her first book was *Natural Hospital Birth: The Best of Both Worlds*. She researches childbirth and parenting cross-culturally in Russia, Canada, the United States, and Brazil. Recent research interests include racial inequalities in childbirth, trauma survivors who give birth, and the cesarean rate in Brazil. She lives and teaches in Ann Arbor, Michigan.

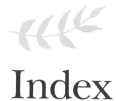

Index

Smoking, 54

Social media, 75

Spacing children, 201–202

Sperlich, Mickey, 193

Starwest Botanicals, 78

"State" cesarean, 193

Steiner, Rudolf, 72

St. John's Wort, 186

Strollers, air travel and, 218

Suicidal thoughts, 189

Suicide hotline, 189

Sunlight exposure, 27, 182, 186

Supplemental nursing/feeding system, 97

Support

    breastfeeding help, 89–93

    by watching baby while you sleep, 57–58

    for emotional well-being, 178–179

    from extended family members, 136,
        140–141

    from partner during first week after child-
        birth, 30–32

    during first week after childbirth, 29, 33

    meal trains, 36–37

    parents giving each other, 30–32

    postpartum depression and, 191

    receiving help from family and friends,
        109–111

    sleep (mother's) and, 63–64

Support groups

    breastfeeding, 92

    finding like-minded mothers at
        mothering, 147

    for new moms, 179–182

Survivor Moms: Women's Stories of Birthing,
    Mothering, and Healing after Sexual Abuse
    (Sperlich/Seng), 193, 196

Swaddling, 22

Sweden, 208

Take Charge of Your Fertility (Weschler), 205

Talk therapy, 183, 185, 191, 196

Technology, limiting use of, 74–75

Testosterone, 17–18

Text-based postpartum depression support
    group, 182

"Thank you," saying to your partner, 114

Therapy, 183, 185, 191, 196

Thompson, Dawn, 194

Tinybeans (online journal), 38

Tongue ties, 90–91

Traumatic birth experiences

    breastfeeding and, 94

    mother's groups and, 179

    postpartum sex and, 168

    PTSD and, 177, 192–194

Travel, 210–220

Tree Town Doulas, 109

Tricyclic antidepressants, 192

Turbin, Kimberly, 194

Twaddle, Tammy, 45

Twilight sleep drugs, 157

Urinating, following childbirth, 23

Urination, baby's, 79–80

Uva ursi leaves, for baths, 77, 78

Vaginal birth

    first two hours after, 19, 20

    when your baby is separated from you, 20

Vaginal bleeding, following birth, 22–23, 203

Vaginal discharge, after birth, 22

Vaginal dryness, 171–172, 203

Vaginal secretions, fertility signs and, 203–204

VBAC (vaginal birth after cesarean), 41

Vernix, 21, 76

Vitamin supplements, 187–188

Weight, birth, 86

Weight gain (baby), 79, 86, 87

Weight loss (baby), 21–22, 27, 86

WIC Peer Counselors, 83

Winnicott, D.W., 70

Women, Infant, and Children (WIC)
    program, 89

Work, returning to

    breastfeeding and, 99–102

    parental leave and, 98–99, 207–208, 209–210

    staying home *versus*, 206–207, 208–209

Worry, sleep and, 62–63

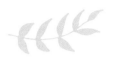

Also Available

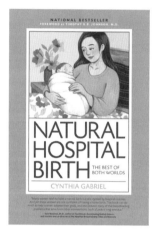

Natural Hospital Birth
978-1-55832-881-5

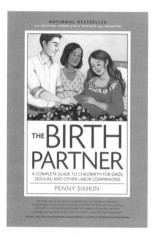

The Birth Partner
978-1-55832-880-8

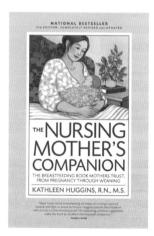

The Nursing Mother's Companion
978-1-55832-882-2